Skill Checklists to Accompany

Taylor's Clinical Nursing Skills:

A NURSING PROCESS APPROACH

Skill Checklists to Accompany

Taylor's Clinical Nursing Skills:

A NURSING PROCESS APPROACH

Pamela Evans-Smith, MSN, FNP
Clinical Nursing Instructor
University of Missouri
Columbia, Missouri

Marilee LeBon, BA
Mountaintop, Pennsylvania

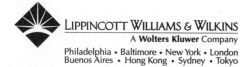
LIPPINCOTT WILLIAMS & WILKINS
A **Wolters Kluwer** Company
Philadelphia • Baltimore • New York • London
Buenos Aires • Hong Kong • Sydney • Tokyo

Developmental Editors: Megan Klim and Claudia Vaughn
Senior Production Editor: Rosanne Hallowell
Director of Nursing Production: Helen Ewan
Managing Editor / Production: Erika Kors
Senior Manufacturing Manager: William Alberti
Compositor: Lippincott Williams & Wilkins
Printer: Victor Graphics

9 8 7 6 5 4 3 2 1

ISBN: 0-7817-5535-2

Care has been taken to confirm the accuracy of the information presented and to describe generally accepted practices. However, the authors, editors, and publisher are not responsible for errors or omissions or for any consequences from application of the information in this book and make no warranty, express or implied, with respect to the content of the publication.

The authors, editors, and publisher have exerted every effort to ensure that drug selection and dosage set forth in this text are in accordance with the current recommendations and practice at the time of publication. However, in view of ongoing research, changes in government regulations, and the constant flow of information relating to drug therapy and drug reactions, the reader is urged to check the package insert for each drug for any change in indications and dosage and for added warnings and precautions This is particularly important when the recommended agent is a new or infrequently employed drug.

Some drugs and medical devices presented in this publication have Food and Drug Administration (FDA) clearance for limited use in restricted research settings. It is the responsibility of the health care provider to ascertain the FDA status of each drug or device planned for use in his or her clinical practice.

LWW.com

Introduction

Developing clinical competency is a major challenge for each fundamentals student. To facilitate the mastery of nursing skills, we are happy to provide Skill Checklists for each procedure in *Taylor Clinical Nursing Skills: A Nursing Process Approach*. The skill checklists follow each step of the procedure to provide a complete evaluative tool. Students can use the checklists to facilitate self-evaluation, and faculty will find them useful in measuring and recording student performance. Three-hole punched and perforated, these checklists can be easily reproduced and brought to the simulation laboratory or clinical area. The checklists are designed to record an evaluation of each step of the procedure.

- Checkmark in the "Excellent" column denotes mastering the procedure.
- Checkmark in the "Satisfactory" column indicates use of the recommended technique.
- Checkmark in the "Needs Practice" column indicates use of *some but not all* of each recommended technique.

The Comments section allows you to highlight suggestions that will improve skills. Space is available at the top of each checklist to record a final pass/fail evaluation, date, and the signature of the student and evaluating faculty member.

List of Skills

x   **Contents**

Skill Checklists to Accompany Taylor's Clinical Nursing Skills:
A Nursing Process Approach

Name _____   Date _____

Unit _____   Position _____

Instructor/Evaluator: _____   Position _____

SKILL 1-1
Assessing a Temperature

Goal: To measure body heat for comparison with accepted normal values.

Excellent	Satisfactory	Needs Practice		Comments
			Assessing Temperature Regardless of Route	
___	___	___	1. Check physician's order or nursing care plan for frequency and route.	
___	___	___	2. Identify patient.	
___	___	___	3. Explain procedure to patient.	
___	___	___	4. Gather equipment.	
___	___	___	5. Make sure the electronic or digital thermometer is in operating condition.	
___	___	___	6. Perform hand hygiene and don gloves if appropriate or indicated.	
___	___	___	7. Select the appropriate site.	
___	___	___	8. Follow steps as outlined below for the appropriate type of thermometer.	
___	___	___	9. Perform hand hygiene. If wearing gloves, discard them in proper receptacle.	
___	___	___	10. Record temperature on paper, flow sheet, or computerized record. Report abnormal findings to the appropriate person. Identify assessment site if other than oral.	
			Assessing Tympanic Membrane Temperature	
___	___	___	1. If necessary, push the "On" button and wait for the "Ready" signal on unit.	
___	___	___	2. Attach tympanic probe cover.	
___	___	___	3. Using gentle but firm pressure, insert probe snugly into external ear, angling thermometer toward patient's jaw line. Pull pinna up and back to staighten the ear canal in an adult.	
___	___	___	4. Activate unit by pushing trigger button. The reading is immediate, usually within 2 seconds. Note temperature reading.	
___	___	___	5. Discard probe cover in appropriate receptacle by pushing the probe release button and replace thermometer in its charger or holder.	

Excellent	Satisfactory	Needs Practice		Comments

Assessing Oral Temperature with an Electronic or Digital Thermometer

1. Release the electronic unit from the charging unit; remove probe from within recording unit.
2. Cover thermometer probe with disposable probe cover; slide it until it snaps into place.
3. Place probe beneath patient's tongue in the posterior sublingual pocket. Ask the patient to close her or his lips around the probe.
4. Continue to hold probe until you hear a beep to let you know the reading is completed. Note the temperature reading.
5. Remove the probe from the patient's mouth and dispose of probe cover by holding probe over appropriate receptacle and pressing probe release button.
6. Return the thermometer probe to the storage place within the unit; return electronic unit to charging unit to make sure it is fully charged.

Assessing Rectal Temperature with an Electronic or Digital Thermometer

1. Put on gloves.
2. Provide privacy for the patient by closing door or curtain.
3. Place the bed at an appropriate working height to reduce back strain during the procedure.
4. Assist the patient into side-lying position. Pull back covers enough to expose only the buttocks.
5. Remove the probe from within the recording unit of the electronic thermometer. Cover the probe with a disposable probe cover and slide it until it snaps into place.
6. Lubricate about 1 inch of the probe with water-soluble lubricant.
7. Reassure patient. Separate the buttocks until anal sphincter is clearly visible.
8. Insert thermometer probe into the anus about 1½ inch in an adult or 1 inch in a child.
9. Hold the probe in place until you hear a beep. Carefully remove the probe. Note the temperature reading on the display.

Excellent	Satisfactory	Needs Practice		Comments

SKILL 1-1
Assessing a Temperature (Continued)

Excellent	Satisfactory	Needs Practice		
___	___	___	10. Dispose of the probe cover by holding probe over appropriate waste receptacle and pressing release button.	
___	___	___	11. Using toilet tissue, wipe the anus of any feces or excess lubricant. Dispose of the toilet tissue.	
___	___	___	12. Remove your gloves and discard. Perform hand hygiene.	
___	___	___	13. Cover the patient and help him or her to a position of comfort. Place bed in lowest position; elevate rails as needed.	
___	___	___	14. Return the thermometer to the charging unit.	

Assessing Axillary Temperature with an Electronic or Digital Thermometer

Excellent	Satisfactory	Needs Practice		
___	___	___	1. Ensure privacy by closing door or curtains.	
___	___	___	2. Place bed at an appropriate working height to reduce back strain during skill.	
___	___	___	3. Move patient's clothing to expose axilla.	
___	___	___	4. Remove probe from recording unit of the electronic thermometer. Slide on a disposable probe cover and snap it securely into place.	
___	___	___	5. Place the end of the probe in the center of the axilla. Have patient bring his or her arm down and close to the body.	
___	___	___	6. Hold the probe in place until you hear a beep, and then carefully remove probe. Note the temperature reading.	
___	___	___	7. Dispose of the probe cover by holding probe over appropriate waste receptacle and pushing release button.	
___	___	___	8. Place the bed in the lowest position and elevate rails as needed. Leave the patient clean and comfortable.	
___	___	___	9. Return the electronic thermometer to the charging unit.	

Assessing Temperature with a Glass Thermometer

Excellent	Satisfactory	Needs Practice		
___	___	___	1. If stored in a chemical solution, wipe thermometer dry with a soft tissue, using a firm twisting motion. Wipe from bulb toward fingers.	
___	___	___	2. Grasp thermometer firmly with the thumb and forefinger. Using strong wrist movements, shake it until the mercury line reaches at least 36°C (59°F).	
___	___	___	3. Read thermometer by holding it horizontally at eye level and rotating it between the fingers until the mercury line is clearly visualized.	

Excellent	Satisfactory	Needs Practice	SKILL 1-1 **Assessing a Temperature** *(Continued)*	Comments
___	___	___	4. Place thermometer's mercury bulb within the back of the right or left pocket under patient's tongue and tell the patient to close lips around thermometer (oral), in the rectum as described when using an electronic thermometer (rectal), or in the center of the axilla with arm against chest wall (axillary).	
___	___	___	5. Leave thermometer in place for 3 minutes or according to agency protocol (oral), 2 to 3 minutes (rectal), and 10 minutes (axillary).	
___	___	___	6. Remove thermometer. Using a firm twisting motion, wipe it once from fingers down to mercury bulb.	
___	___	___	7. Dispose of tissues in a receptacle for contaminated items.	
___	___	___	8. Read thermometer to nearest tenth.	
___	___	___	9. Wash thermometer in lukewarm soapy water. Rinse it in cool water. Dry and replace thermometer in its container.	

Skill Checklists to Accompany Taylor's Clinical Nursing Skills:
A Nursing Process Approach

Name _____ Date _____

Unit _____ Position _____

Instructor/Evaluator: _____ Position _____

Excellent	Satisfactory	Needs Practice	SKILL 1-2 **Assessing a Pulse**	Comments
			Goal: To measure heart rate for comparison with accepted normal values while causing no trauma to the patient.	
___	___	___	1. Identify patient.	
___	___	___	2. Explain procedure to patient.	
___	___	___	3. Gather equipment.	
___	___	___	4. Perform hand hygiene and don gloves as appropriate.	
___	___	___	5. Select appropriate site.	
___	___	___	6. Follow steps as outlined below for appropriate pulse assessment.	
___	___	___	7. Perform hand hygiene.	
___	___	___	8. Record pulse rate and site on paper, flow sheet, or computerized record. Report abnormal findings to appropriate person. Identify assessment site if other than apical.	
			Palpating the Radial Pulse	
___	___	___	1. Patient may either be supine with arm alongside body, wrist extended, and palms lateral or facing down or sitting with forearm at a 90-degree angle to body resting on a support with wrist extended and palm downward or facing laterally.	
___	___	___	2. Place your first, second, and third fingers along patient's radial artery and press gently against the radius. Rest your thumb on back of patient's wrist.	
___	___	___	3. Apply only enough pressure to distinctly feel the artery.	
___	___	___	4. Using a watch with a second hand, count the number of pulsations felt for 30 seconds. Multiply this number by 2 to have rate for 1 minute. If pulse's rate, rhythm, or amplitude are abnormal in any way, palpate for 1 minute longer.	
			Auscultating the Apical Pulse Rate	
___	___	___	1. Use alcohol swab to clean stethoscope ear pieces and diaphragm.	

Excellent	Satisfactory	Needs Practice				SKILL 1-2 **Assessing a Pulse** (*Continued*)	Comments

SKILL 1-2

Assessing a Pulse (*Continued*)

Excellent	Satisfactory	Needs Practice		Comments
⎯	⎯	⎯	2. Assist patient to sit in chair or sit up in bed and then expose chest area.	
⎯	⎯	⎯	3. Hold stethoscope diaphragm against the palm of your hand for a few seconds.	
⎯	⎯	⎯	4. Palpate the fifth intercostal space and move to left midclavicular line. Place diaphragm over apex of the heart.	
⎯	⎯	⎯	5. Listen for heart sounds, identified as a "lub-dub" sound.	
⎯	⎯	⎯	6. Using watch with a second hand, count heartbeat for 1 minute.	
			Using a Doppler to Assess the Pulse Rate	
⎯	⎯	⎯	1. Remove Doppler from charger and turn on. Make sure that volume is low.	
⎯	⎯	⎯	2. Apply Doppler gel to the site where you are auscultating the pulse.	
⎯	⎯	⎯	3. Hold the Doppler in your nondominant hand. Using your dominant hand, place the Doppler tip in the gel. Adjust the volume as needed. Move the Doppler tip around until the pulse is heard.	
⎯	⎯	⎯	4. Using a watch with a second hand, count the heartbeat for 1 minute.	
⎯	⎯	⎯	5. Remove the Doppler tip and turn the Doppler off. Wipe the gel off of the patient's extremity with tissue.	
⎯	⎯	⎯	6. Return the Doppler to the charge base.	

Skill Checklists to Accompany Taylor's Clinical Nursing Skills:
A Nursing Process Approach

Name _____ Date _____

Unit _____ Position _____

Instructor/Evaluator: _____ Position _____

Excellent	Satisfactory	Needs Practice	SKILL 1-3 **Assessing Respiration**	Comments
			Goal: To measure pulmonary ventilation for comparison with accepted normal values while causing no trauma to the patient.	
___	___	___	1. While your fingers are still in place after counting the pulse rate, observe patient's respirations.	
___	___	___	2. Note rise and fall of patient's chest.	
___	___	___	3. Using a watch with a second hand, count number of respirations for a minimum of 30 seconds. Multiply this number by 2 for respiratory rate per minute.	
___	___	___	4. If respirations are abnormal in any way, count respirations for at least 1 full minute.	
___	___	___	5. Perform hand hygiene.	
___	___	___	6. Document respiratory rate on paper, flow sheet, or computerized record. Report any abnormal findings to appropriate person.	

Skill Checklists to Accompany Taylor's Clinical Nursing Skills:
A Nursing Process Approach

Name _____   Date _____

Unit _____   Position _____

Instructor/Evaluator: _____   Position _____

SKILL 1-4
Assessing a Blood Pressure

Goal: To measure force of blood against arterial walls for comparison with accepted normal values while causing no trauma to the patient.

Excellent	Satisfactory	Needs Practice		Comments
___	___	___	1. Identify the patient.	
___	___	___	2. Explain procedure to patient.	
___	___	___	3. Gather equipment.	
___	___	___	4. Perform hand hygiene.	
___	___	___	5. Delay obtaining the blood pressure if the patient is emotionally upset, is in pain, or has just exercised, unless it is urgent to obtain blood pressure.	
___	___	___	6. Select appropriate arm for application of cuff (no intravenous infusion, breast, or axilla surgery on that side; cast arteriovenous shunt; or injured or diseased limb).	
___	___	___	7. Have patient assume a comfortable lying or sitting position with forearm supported at the level of the heart and with palm upward.	
___	___	___	8. Expose area of brachial artery by removing garments or moving sleeve, if it is not too tight, above area where cuff will be placed.	
___	___	___	9. Center the bladder of the cuff over brachial artery approximately midway on arm, so lower edge of cuff is about 2.5 to 5 cm (1 to 2 inches) above the inner aspect of the elbow. Tubing should extend from cuff edge nearer patient's elbow.	
___	___	___	10. Wrap cuff smoothly and snugly around the arm. Fasten it securely or tuck end of cuff well under preceding wrapping. Do not allow any clothing to interfere with proper placement of cuff.	
___	___	___	11. Check that the needle on the aneroid gauge is within the zero mark. If using a mercury manometer, check to see that the manometer is in a vertical position and that the mercury is within the zero level with the gauge at eye level.	
___	___	___	12. Palpate the pulse at the brachial or radial artery by pressing gently with the fingertips.	

Excellent	Satisfactory	Needs Practice	SKILL 1-4 **Assessing a Blood Pressure** *(Continued)*	Comments
——	——	——	13. Tighten the screw valve on the air pump.	
——	——	——	14. Inflate the cuff while continuing to palpate the artery. Note the point on the gauge where the pulse disappears.	
——	——	——	15. Deflate the cuff and wait 15 seconds.	
——	——	——	16. Assume a position that is no more than 3 feet away from the gauge.	
——	——	——	17. Place the stethoscope earpieces in the ears. Direct the ear tips forward into the canal and not against the ear itself.	
——	——	——	18. Place the stethoscope bell or diaphragm firmly but with as little pressure as possible over the brachial artery. Do not allow stethoscope to touch clothing or cuff.	
——	——	——	19. Pump the pressure 30 mm Hg above the point at which the systolic pressure was palpated and estimated. Open manometer valve and allow air to escape slowly (allowing gauge to drop 2 to 3 mm per heartbeat).	
——	——	——	20. Note the point on the gauge at which the first faint, but clear, sound appears and slowly increases in intensity. Note this number as the systolic pressure.	
——	——	——	21. Read pressure to the closest even number.	
——	——	——	22. Do not reinflate cuff once air is being released to recheck the systolic pressure reading.	
——	——	——	23. Note the pressure at which the sound first becomes muffled. Also observe point at which sound completely disappears. These may occur separately or at the same point.	
——	——	——	24. Allow remaining air to escape quickly. Repeat any suspicious reading but wait 30 to 60 seconds between readings to allow normal circulation to return to limb. Be sure to deflate cuff completely between attempts to check blood pressure.	
——	——	——	25. Remove cuff. Clean and store equipment.	
——	——	——	26. Perform hand hygiene. If gloves are worn, discard them in the proper receptacle.	
——	——	——	27. Record the findings on paper flow sheet or computerized record. Report abnormal findings to the appropriate person. Identify arm used and site of assessment if other than brachial.	

SKILL 1-4
Assessing a Blood Pressure *(Continued)*

Excellent	Satisfactory	Needs Practice		Comments

Assessing Blood Pressure with an Electric Device

Follow Actions 1 to 10 above, then:

11. Turn the machine on. If the machine has different setting for an infant, child, or adult, make sure that the appropriate setting is selected. Push start. Instruct the patient to hold arm still.

12. Wait until the machine beeps and blood pressure reading appears. Remove the cuff from the patient's arm; clean and store the equipment.

13. Perform hand hygiene. If gloves are worn, discard them in the proper receptacle.

14. Record the findings on paper, flow sheet, or computerized record. Report abnormal findings to the appropriate person. Identify arm used and site of assessment if other than brachial.

Using a Doppler Ultrasound to Measure Blood Pressure

Follow Actions 1 to 11 above, then:

12. Place a small amount of gel over the brachial artery.

13. Hold the Doppler in your nondominant hand. Using your dominant hand, place the Doppler tip in the gel. Adjust the volume as needed. Move the Doppler tip around until the pulse is heard.

14. Once the pulse is found using the Doppler, close valve to sphygmomanometer. Tighten the screw valve on the air pump.

15. Inflate the cuff while continuing to use the Doppler on the artery. Note the point on the gauge where the pulse disappears.

16. Allow the remaining air to escape quickly. Repeat any suspicious reading but wait 30 to 60 seconds between readings to allow normal circulation to return in the limb. Be sure to deflate the cuff completely between attempts to check the blood pressure.

17. Remove the cuff, and clean and store the equipment.

18. Perform hand hygiene. If gloves are worn, discard them in the proper receptacle.

19. Record the findings on paper, flow sheet, or computerized record. Report abnormal findings to the appropriate person. Identify arm used and site of assessment if other than brachial.

Skill Checklists to Accompany Taylor's Clinical Nursing Skills:
A Nursing Process Approach

Name _____   Date _____

Unit _____   Position _____

Instructor/Evaluator: _____   Position _____

Excellent	Satisfactory	Needs Practice	SKILL 1-5 **Using a Bedscale**	Comments
			Goal: To achieve an accurate weight measurement using the bedscale while keeping the patient safe from injury.	
____	____	____	1. Identify the patient.	
____	____	____	2. Explain the procedure to the patient.	
____	____	____	3. Gather equipment.	
____	____	____	4. Perform hand hygiene.	
____	____	____	5. Unplug the bedscale from electrical outlet. Slide disposable plastic cover over the sling of the bedscale.	
____	____	____	6. Attach the sling to the bedscale. Turn the scale on. Adjust the dial so that weight is now 0.0.	
____	____	____	7. Remove the sling from the scale. Raise bed to a comfortable working level. Roll sling long ways. Raise side rail. Turn patient onto side facing side rail. Place rolled sling under patient.	
____	____	____	8. Roll patient back over sling and up on other side. Pull sling through (as if placing sheet under patient).	
____	____	____	9. Roll scale so that arms of scale are directly over patient. Spread the base of the scale. Remove pillow and blankets. Lower arms of the scale and place hooks into holes on the sling.	
____	____	____	10. Once scale arms are hooked onto the sling, begin to crank scale so that patient is lifted up off of the bed. Assess all tubes and drains, making sure that none has tension placed on them as the scale is lifted. Once the sling is free from touching the bed, ensure that nothing else is hanging onto the sling (eg, ventilator tubing, intravenous tubing, etc.). If any tubing is connected to the patient, raise it up so that it is not adding any weight to the patient.	
____	____	____	11. Note weight on the scale. Slowly lower patient gently back onto bed. Disconnect scale arms from sling. Close base of scale and remove from patient's room.	
____	____	____	12. Raise side rail. Turn patient to side rail. Roll the sling up against the patient's backside.	
____	____	____	13. Raise the other side rail. Roll patient back over the sling and up facing the other side rail. Remove sling from bed.	

Excellent	Satisfactory	Needs Practice	SKILL 1-5 **Using a Bedscale** (*Continued*)	Comments
___	___	___	14. Position patient into comfortable position. Lower the bed.	
___	___	___	15. Remove disposable cover from sling and discard in appropriate receptacle. Replace scale and sling in appropriate spot. Plug scale into electrical outlet.	
___	___	___	16. Document weight and scale used.	

Skill Checklists to Accompany Taylor's Clinical Nursing Skills:
A Nursing Process Approach

Name _____ Date _____

Unit _____ Position _____

Instructor/Evaluator: _____ Position _____

SKILL 1-6
Monitoring Temperature Using Overhead Radiant Warmer

Goal: To measure temperature of infant when using an overhead warmer to control temperature and to ensure that the infant experiences no injury.

Excellent	Satisfactory	Needs Practice		Comments
___	___	___	1. Identify the patient.	
___	___	___	2. Explain the procedure to the family.	
___	___	___	3. Gather equipment.	
___	___	___	4. Perform hand hygiene.	
___	___	___	5. Plug the warmer in. Turn the warmer onto manual setting. Allow the blankets to warm before placing the infant under the warmer.	
___	___	___	6. Switch the warmer setting to automatic. Place the infant under the warmer. Attach probe to the infant so that the probe is directly under the radiant heaters but not on a bony area. Cover with a foil patch.	
___	___	___	7. Adjust the temperature as ordered.	
___	___	___	8. Continue to monitor the infant's axillary temperature as ordered. The temperature may need to be monitored more frequently in the beginning.	
___	___	___	9. Adjust the warmer's temperature as needed according to the axillary temperatures.	
___	___	___	10. Document the placement of the infant under the radiant warmer and the settings of the radiant warmer.	

Skill Checklists to Accompany Taylor's Clinical Nursing Skills:
A Nursing Process Approach

Name _____   Date _____

Unit _____   Position _____

Instructor/Evaluator: _____   Position _____

SKILL 2-1
Performing a Head-to-Toe Physical Assessment

Goal: To perform an assessment in which the patient participates and demonstrates a decrease in anxiety level related to assessment and possible findings.

Excellent	Satisfactory	Needs Practice		Comments
____	____	____	1. Explain the physical examination and answer questions.	
____	____	____	2. Instruct the patient to void if possible. Collect a urine specimen if ordered.	
____	____	____	3. Perform hand hygiene.	
____	____	____	4. Help the patient undress and provide a gown.	
____	____	____	5. Measure and record height, weight, and vital signs.	
____	____	____	6. Assist the patient onto the examination table, stretcher, or bed; position and drape the patient according to body area to be assessed.	
____	____	____	7. Perform a physical examination, starting at the head and working in a systematic fashion. Don gloves when indicated.	
____	____	____	8. Inspect the head, noting hair color, texture, and distribution. Palpate from the forehead to the posterior triangle of the neck for the posterior cervical lymph nodes.	
____	____	____	9. Palpate in front of and behind the ears, under the chin, and in the anterior triangle for the anterior cervical lymph nodes.	
____	____	____	10. Palpate the left and then the right carotid arteries and auscultate the arteries.	
____	____	____	11. Palpate the trachea and then the suprasternal notch.	
____	____	____	12. Palpate the supraclavicular area.	
____	____	____	13. Palpate and then auscultate the thyroid gland.	
____	____	____	14. Have the patient touch his or her chin to chest and to each shoulder, each ear to the corresponding shoulder, and then tip head back as far as possible.	
____	____	____	15. Place your hands on the patient's shoulders while he or she shrugs them against resistance; then place your hand on the patient's left cheek and then the right cheek and have the patient push against it.	
____	____	____	16. Have the patient smile, frown, wrinkle forehead, and puff out cheeks.	

Excellent	Satisfactory	Needs Practice	SKILL 2-1 **Performing a Head-to-Toe Physical Assessment** *(Continued)*
			Comments
——	——	——	17. Occlude one nostril externally with a finger while patient breathes through the other; repeat for the other side.
——	——	——	18. Inspect the internal nostrils using an otoscope with a nasal speculum attachment or an ophthalmoscope handle with a nasal attachment.
——	——	——	19. Palpate the nose and then palpate and percuss the frontal and maxillary sinuses. Transilluminate the sinuses if the patient complains of tenderness.
——	——	——	20. Palpate the temporomandibular joint as the patient opens and closes the jaw.
——	——	——	21. Inspect the oral mucosa, gingivae, teeth, and salivary gland openings using a tongue blade and penlight.
——	——	——	22. Observe the tongue and hard and soft palates. Ask the patient to stick out his or her tongue; ask the patient to say "ah" while sticking out the tongue. Inspect the visible oral structures.
——	——	——	23. Test the gag reflex.
——	——	——	24. Place a tongue blade at the side of the tongue while patient pushes it to the left and right with the tongue.
——	——	——	25. Ask the patient to close the eyes and identify the smell of different substances such as coffee, chocolate, alcohol, or other known substances.
——	——	——	26. Test the patient's visual acuity with a Snellen chart or another chart; have the patient identify the pattern in a specially prepared page of color dots or plates.
——	——	——	27. Move the patient's eyes through the six cardinal positions of gaze.
——	——	——	28. Inspect the external eye structures, conjunctiva, and sclera.
——	——	——	29. Inspect the cornea, iris, and anterior chamber by shining a penlight tangentially across the eye.
——	——	——	30. Examine the pupils for equality of size, shape, reaction to light, and accommodation.
——	——	——	31. Using an ophthalmoscope, check the red reflex.
——	——	——	32. Inspect the ear and perform an otoscopic examination; palpate the ear and mastoid process.
——	——	——	33. Use a whispered voice or ticking of watch to test hearing, one ear at a time.
——	——	——	34. Use a tuning fork to perform Weber's test and Rinne's test.

Excellent	Satisfactory	Needs Practice	SKILL 2-1 **Performing a Head-to-Toe** **Physical Assessment** *(Continued)*	
				Comments
⎯	⎯	⎯	35. Inspect the posterior thorax. Observe the skin, bones, and muscles of the spine, shoulder blades, and back as well as symmetry of expansion and accessory muscle use.	
⎯	⎯	⎯	36. Assess anteroposterior and lateral diameters of the thorax.	
⎯	⎯	⎯	37. Palpate over the spine and posterior thorax.	
⎯	⎯	⎯	38. Assess respiratory excursion and tactile fremitus (as the patient repeats the word "ninety-nine").	
⎯	⎯	⎯	39. Percuss over the posterior and lateral lung fields and for diaphragmatic excursion on each side of the thorax.	
⎯	⎯	⎯	40. Auscultate the lungs through the posterior thorax as the patient breathes slowly and deeply through the mouth.	
⎯	⎯	⎯	41. Examine the anterior thorax. Observe the skin, bones, and muscles as well as symmetry of expansion and accessory muscle use.	
⎯	⎯	⎯	42. Inspect the anterior thorax for lifts, heaves, or thrusts; check for the apical impulse; palpate over the anterior thorax.	
⎯	⎯	⎯	43. Assess respiratory excursion and tactile fremitus (as the patient repeats the word "ninety-nine").	
⎯	⎯	⎯	44. Percuss over the anterior thorax.	
⎯	⎯	⎯	45. Auscultate the lungs through the anterior thorax as the patient breathes slowly and deeply through the mouth.	
⎯	⎯	⎯	46. Inspect the breasts and axillae with the patient's hands resting on both sides of the body, placed on the hips, and then raised above the head.	
⎯	⎯	⎯	47. Palpate the axillae with the patient's arms resting against the side of the body; palpate the breasts and nipples with the patient lying supine.	
⎯	⎯	⎯	48. Inspect the neck for jugular vein distention with patient lying supine with head of bed raised to a 45-degree angle.	
⎯	⎯	⎯	49. Palpate the precordium for the apical impulse; auscultate the aortic, pulmonic, Erb's point, tricuspid, and mitral areas for heart sounds.	
⎯	⎯	⎯	50. Assess the abdomen by observing contour, inspecting for skin characteristics, symmetry, contour, peristalsis, and pulsations.	
⎯	⎯	⎯	51. Visualize the four quadrants. Auscultate all four quadrants before percussing or palpating.	

Excellent	Satisfactory	Needs Practice		Comments
			SKILL 2-1 **Performing a Head-to-Toe** **Physical Assessment** *(Continued)*	
____	____	____	52. Percuss from below the right breast to the inguinal area down the right midclavicular line; percuss in a similar fashion on the left; percuss the area over the symphysis pubis.	
____	____	____	53. Palpate all four abdominal quadrants.	
____	____	____	54. Palpate for the kidneys on each side of the abdomen; palpate the liver at the right costal border; palpate for the spleen at the left costal border. If the patient complains of abdominal pain, assess for rebound tenderness last by palpating deeply in the area of the pain and then releasing suddenly. If positive, avoid continued palpation of the abdomen.	
____	____	____	55. Palpate and auscultate the femoral pulses in the groin.	
____	____	____	56. Inspect the external genitalia and rectal area. Have client hold his penis after inspection.	
____	____	____	57. Examine the arms. Observe the skin and muscle mass.	
____	____	____	58. Ask patient to extend arms forward and then rapidly turn palms up and down.	
____	____	____	59. Place your hands on patient's upturned forearms while the patient pushes up against resistance and then place your hands under the forearms while patient pushes down.	
____	____	____	60. Inspect and palpate the fingers, wrists, and elbow joints; palpate the patient's hands. Check skin turgor.	
____	____	____	61. Palpate the radial and brachial pulses.	
____	____	____	62. Inspect the color, shape, and condition of patient's nails; check for capillary refill.	
____	____	____	63. Have the patient squeeze two of your fingers placed in the palm of the hand.	
____	____	____	64. Examine the legs. Inspect the legs and feet for color, lesions, varicosities, hair growth, nail growth, edema, and muscle mass.	
____	____	____	65. Test for pitting edema in the pretibial area.	
____	____	____	66. Palpate for pulses and skin temperature at the posterior tibial, dorsalis pedis, and popliteal areas.	
____	____	____	67. Have the patient perform the straight leg test, one leg at a time.	
____	____	____	68. Palpate for crepitus as the patient abducts and adducts the hip; repeat on the other side.	
____	____	____	69. Ask the patient to raise his or her thigh against the resistance of your hand; next have the patient push	

Excellent	Satisfactory	Needs Practice		Comments

outward against the resistance of your hand and then have the patient pull backward against the resistance of your hands. Repeat on the opposite side.

70. Assess the patient's deep tendon reflexes.

   a. Place fingers above the patient's wrist and tap them with a reflex hammer; repeat on the other arm.

   b. Place fingers over the antecubital area and tap with a reflex hammer; repeat on the other side.

   c. Place fingers over the triceps tendon area and tape with a reflex hammer; repeat on the other side.

   d. Tap just below the patella with a reflex hammer; repeat on the other side.

   e. Tap over the Achilles tendon area with reflex hammer; repeat on the other side.

71. Stroke the sole of the patient's foot with the end of a reflex hammer handle or other hard objects such as a key; repeat on the other side.

72. Ask patient to dorsiflex and then plantar flex both feet against resistance.

73. Using your finger or applicator, trace a one-digit number on the patient's palm and ask to identify the number. Place a familiar object such as key in the patient's hand and ask to identify the object.

74. Observe the patient as he or she walks with a regular gait, on the toes, on the heels, and then heel-to-toe.

75. Perform Romberg's test; ask the patient to stand straight with both eyes closed and both arms extended with palms up.

76. Document significant normal and abnormal findings in an organized manner according to the related body systems.

Skill Checklists to Accompany Taylor's Clinical Nursing Skills:
A Nursing Process Approach

Name _____   Date _____

Unit _____   Position _____

Instructor/Evaluator: _____   Position _____

Excellent	Satisfactory	Needs Practice	SKILL 2-2 **Collecting a Venous Blood Sample by Venipuncture** **Goal:** To obtain a specimen without the patient experiencing undue anxiety and injury.	Comments
____	____	____	1. Gather the necessary supplies. If you are using evacuated tubes (Vacutainer), open the needle packet, attach the needle to its holder, and select the appropriate tubes. If you are using a syringe, attach the appropriate needle to it. Be sure to choose a syringe large enough to hold all the blood required for the test. Label all collection tubes clearly with the patient's name and room number, the physician's name, the date and time of collection, and your initials (since you will be the person performing the venipuncture).	
____	____	____	2. Perform hand hygiene and put on gloves.	
____	____	____	3. Confirm the patient's identity and tell him that you are about to collect a blood sample; explain the procedure to ease anxiety and ensure cooperation. Ask him if he has ever felt faint, sweaty, or nauseated when having blood drawn.	
____	____	____	4. If the patient is on bed rest, ask him to lie in a supine position, with his head slightly elevated and his arms at his sides. Ask the ambulatory patient to sit in a chair and support his arm securely on an armrest or a table.	
____	____	____	5. Assess the patient's veins to determine the best puncture site. Observe the skin for the vein's blue color or palpate the vein for a firm rebound sensation.	
____	____	____	6. Tie a tourniquet 5 cm proximal to the area chosen by pulling the ends tightly in the opposite directions. Tuck one end beneath the other.	
____	____	____	7. If the tourniquet fails to dilate the vein, have the patient open and close his fist a few times. Then ask him to close his fist as you insert the needle and to open it again when the needle is in place.	
____	____	____	8. Clean the venipuncture site with an antimicrobial swab per agency policy, wiping in a circular motion spiraling outward. If using alcohol, apply it with friction for 30 seconds or until the final pad comes away clean. Allow the skin to dry before performing the venipuncture.	

Excellent	Satisfactory	Needs Practice	SKILL 2-2 **Collecting a Venous Blood Sample by Venipuncture** (Continued)	
				Comments
___	___	___	9. Press just below the venipuncture site with your thumb and drawing the skin taut.	
___	___	___	10. Position the needle holder or syringe with the needle bevel up and the shaft parallel to the path of the vein and at a 30-degree angle to the arm. Insert the needle into the vein.	
___	___	___	a. If using a syringe, look for venous blood to appear in the hub; withdraw the blood slowly, pulling the plunger of the syringe gently to create steady suction until you obtain the required sample.	
___	___	___	b. If using a needle holder and an evacuated tube, grasp the holder securely to stabilize it in the vein and push down on the collection tube until the needle punctures the rubber stopper. Blood will flow into the tube automatically.	
___	___	___	11. Remove the tourniquet as soon as blood flows adequately.	
___	___	___	12. Continue to fill the required tubes, removing one and inserting another. Gently rotate each tube as you remove it.	
___	___	___	13. After you have drawn the sample, place a gauze pad over the puncture site and slowly and gently remove the needle from the vein. When using an evacuated tube, remove the specimen tube from the needle holder to release the vacuum before withdrawing the needle from the vein.	
___	___	___	14. Apply gentle pressure to the puncture site for 2 to 3 minutes or until bleeding stops.	
___	___	___	15. After bleeding stops, apply an adhesive bandage.	
___	___	___	16. If you have used a syringe, transfer the sample to a collection tube.	
___	___	___	17. Place the specimen tubes inside the biohazard transport bag and handle carefully avoid foaming.	
___	___	___	18. Check the venipuncture site to see if a hematoma has developed.	
___	___	___	19. Discard syringes, needles, and used gloves in the appropriate containers. Perform hand hygiene.	
___	___	___	20. Record the date, time, and site of the venipuncture; the name of the test; the time the sample was sent to the laboratory; the amount of blood collected; the patient's temperature; and any adverse reactions to the procedure.	

Skill Checklists to Accompany Taylor's Clinical Nursing Skills:
A Nursing Process Approach

Name _____   Date _____

Unit _____   Position _____

Instructor/Evaluator: _____   Position _____

SKILL 2-3
Obtaining a Blood Specimen for Culture and Sensitivity

Goal: To obtain a specimen without the patient experiencing undue anxiety and injury.

Excellent	Satisfactory	Needs Practice		Comments
___	___	___	1. Tell the patient that you need to collect a series of blood samples to check for infection. Explain the procedure, including that the procedure usually requires three blood samples collected at different times.	
___	___	___	2. Perform hand hygiene and put on gloves.	
___	___	___	3. Tie a tourniquet 29 (5 cm) proximal to the area chosen, clean the site with an alcohol or a povidone-iodine pad, and perform the venipuncture (see Skill 2-2).	
___	___	___	4. Withdraw approximately 10 mL of blood from an adult and complete the venipuncture.	
___	___	___	5. Wipe the diaphragm tops of the culture bottles with a povidone-iodine pad and allow to dry.	
___	___	___	6. Change the needle on the syringe used to draw the blood. Then inject 5 mL of blood into each bottle.	
___	___	___	7. Label the culture bottles with the patient's name and room number, physician's name, and date and time of collection. Indicate the suspected diagnosis and the patient's temperature and note on the laboratory request form any recent antibiotic therapy.	
___	___	___	8. Place the samples in the laboratory biohazard transport bag and send the samples to the laboratory immediately.	
___	___	___	9. Discard syringes, needles, and gloves in the appropriate containers. Perform hand hygiene and record the date and time of blood sample collection, name of the test, amount of blood collected, number of bottles used, patient's temperature, and adverse reactions to the procedure.	

Skill Checklists to Accompany Taylor's Clinical Nursing Skills:
A Nursing Process Approach

Name _____   Date _____

Unit _____   Position _____

Instructor/Evaluator: _____   Position _____

SKILL 3-1
Applying Cloth Restraint to an Extremity

Goal: To contain patient by the cloth restraint without interfering with his or her lines, dressings, or other equipment and without causing injury to the patient.

Excellent	Satisfactory	Needs Practice		Comments
___	___	___	1. Determine the need for restraints. Assess patient's physical condition, behavior, and mental status.	
___	___	___	2. Confirm agency policy for application of restraints. Secure a physician's order and ensure that physician's order has been obtained within the past 24 hours.	
___	___	___	3. Explain reason for use to patient and family. Clarify how care will be given and needs will be met. Reinforce the explanation that use of restraint is a temporary measure.	
___	___	___	4. Perform hand hygiene.	
___	___	___	5. Apply restraints according to manufacturer's direction.	
___	___	___	a. Choose the least restrictive type of device that allows the greatest possible degree of mobility.	
___	___	___	b. Pad bony prominences.	
___	___	___	c. For restraint applied to extremity, ensure that two fingers can be inserted between the restraint and patient's wrist or ankle. If the restraint is applied around the torso or abdomen, a hand or fist should fit under the restraint. Maintain restrained extremity in normal anatomic position.	
___	___	___	d. Use appropriate tie for all restraints.	
___	___	___	e. Fasten restraint to the bed frame and not the side rail. Site should not be readily accessible to the patient.	
___	___	___	6. Remove restraint at least every 2 hours or according to agency policy and patient need.	
___	___	___	a. Check for signs of decreased circulation or impaired skin integrity.	
___	___	___	b. Perform range-of-motion exercises before reapplying restraint.	
___	___	___	7. Reassure patient at regular intervals. Store call bell within easy reach.	
___	___	___	8. Assess for signs of sensory deprivation, such as increased sleeping, daydreaming, anxiety, panic, and hallucinations.	

SKILL 3-1

Applying Cloth Restraint to an Extremity *(Continued)*

Excellent	Satisfactory	Needs Practice		Comments
——	——	——	9. Perform hand hygiene.	
——	——	——	10. Document reason for restraining patient, alternative measures attempted before applying the restraint, date and time of application, type of restraint, times when removed, and result and frequency of nursing assessment every 2 hours. Obtain a new order after 24 hours if restraints are still necessary.	

Name _____ Date _____

Unit _____ Position _____

Instructor/Evaluator: _____ Position _____

Excellent	Satisfactory	Needs Practice	SKILL 3-2 **Applying a Vest Restraint**	Comments
			Goal: To contain a patient by a vest restraint to prevent him or her from falling.	
___	___	___	1. Determine the need for restraints. Assess patient's physical condition, behavior, and mental status.	
___	___	___	2. Confirm agency policy for application of restraints. Secure a physician's order. Ensure that physician's order has been obtained within the past 24 hours.	
___	___	___	3. Explain reason for use to patient and family. Clarify how care will be given and needs will be met and that use of restraint is a temporary measure.	
___	___	___	4. Perform hand hygiene.	
___	___	___	5. Apply restraints according to manufacturer's direction.	
___	___	___	a. Choose the correct size of the least restrictive type of device that allows the greatest possible degree of mobility.	
___	___	___	b. Pad bony prominences or therapeutic devices that may be affected by the vest.	
___	___	___	c. Assist patient to a sitting position, if not contraindicated.	
___	___	___	d. Place vest on patient, over gown, with flaps crisscrossing over the patient's abdomen if appropriate. The V opening should be on the front of the patient.	
___	___	___	e. Pull the tabs secure. Ensure there are no wrinkles in the vest behind patient.	
___	___	___	f. Insert fist between the restraint and patient to ensure that breathing is not constricted. Assess respirations after restraint is applied.	
___	___	___	g. Use appropriate tie for all restraints.	
___	___	___	h. Fasten restraint to the bed frame and not the side rail. Place bed height in low position. If patient is in a wheelchair, lock the wheels and place the restraints under the arm rests and tie behind the chair. Site should not be readily accessible to the patient.	

Excellent	Satisfactory	Needs Practice	SKILL 3-2 **Applying a Vest Restraint** *(Continued)*	Comments
——	——	——	6. Remove restraint at least every 2 hours or according to agency policy and patient need. Check for any signs of respiratory difficulties.	
——	——	——	7. Reassure patient at regular intervals. Store call bell within easy reach.	
——	——	——	8. Assess for signs of sensory deprivation, such as increased sleeping, daydreaming, anxiety, panic, and hallucinations.	
——	——	——	9. Perform hand hygiene.	
——	——	——	10. Document reason for restraining patient, alternative measures attempted before applying the restraint, date and time of application, type of restraint, times when removed, and result and frequency of nursing assessment every 2 hours. Obtain a new order after 24 hours if restraints are still necessary.	

Skill Checklists to Accompany Taylor's Clinical Nursing Skills:
A Nursing Process Approach

Name _____   Date _____

Unit _____   Position _____

Instructor/Evaluator: _____   Position _____

Excellent	Satisfactory	Needs Practice	SKILL 3-3 **Applying an Elbow Restraint**	Comments
			Goal: To prevent a patient from reaching and interfering with dressings, incisions, or therapeutic devices without causing harm to the patient.	
___	___	___	1. Determine the need for restraints. Assess patient's physical condition, behavior, and mental status.	
___	___	___	2. Confirm agency policy for application of restraints. Secure a physician's order. Ensure that physician's order has been obtained within the past 24 hours.	
___	___	___	3. Explain reason for use to patient and family. Clarify how care will be given and needs will be met and that use of restraint is a temporary measure.	
___	___	___	4. Perform hand hygiene.	
___	___	___	5. Apply restraints according to manufacturer's direction.	
___	___	___	a. Choose the least restrictive type of device that allows the greatest possible degree of mobility.	
___	___	___	b. Pad bony prominences. If patient has infusion or dressing on arm, extra padding may be applied.	
___	___	___	c. Spread elbow restraint out flat. Place middle of elbow restraint behind patient's elbow. The restraint should not extend below the wrist or place pressure on the axilla.	
___	___	___	d. Wrap snugly around the patient's arm, but ensure that two fingers can easily fit under the restraint.	
___	___	___	e. Wrap Velcro straps around the elbow restraint.	
___	___	___	f. Apply other elbow restraint to opposite arm if patient can move arm.	
___	___	___	g. Thread Velcro strap from one elbow restraint across the back and into the loop on the opposite elbow restraint.	
___	___	___	h. Assess circulation to the fingers and hand.	
___	___	___	6. Remove restraint at least every 2 hours or according to agency policy and patient need.	
___	___	___	a. Check for signs of decreased circulation or impaired skin integrity.	
___	___	___	b. Perform range of motion exercises before reapplying.	

Excellent	Satisfactory	Needs Practice		Comments

SKILL 3-3

Applying an Elbow Restraint *(Continued)*

7. Reassure patient at regular intervals. Store call bell within easy reach.

8. Assess for signs of sensory deprivation, such as increased sleeping, daydreaming, anxiety, inconsolable crying, and panic.

9. Perform hand hygiene.

10. Document reason for restraining patient, alternative measures attempted before applying the restraint, date and time of application, type of restraint, times when removed, and result and frequency of nursing assessment every 2 hours. Obtain a new order after 24 hours if restraints are still necessary.

28

Name _____   Date _____

Unit _____   Position _____

Instructor/Evaluator: _____   Position _____

Excellent	Satisfactory	Needs Practice	SKILL 3-4 **Applying Leather Restraints**	Comments
			Goal: To contain a patient using a leather restraint without the patient causing harm to self or others.	
___	___	___	1. Determine the need for restraints. Assess patient's physical condition, behavior, and mental status.	
___	___	___	2. Confirm agency policy for application of restraints. Secure a physician's order. Ensure that physician's order has been obtained within the past 24 hours.	
___	___	___	3. Explain reason for use to patient and family. Clarify how care will be given and needs will be met and that use of restraint is a temporary measure.	
___	___	___	4. Perform hand hygiene.	
___	___	___	5. Apply restraints according to manufacturer's direction.	
___	___	___	a. Pad bony prominences.	
___	___	___	b. For restraint applied to extremity, ensure that two fingers can be inserted between the restraint and patient's wrist or ankle.	
___	___	___	c. Maintain restrained extremity in normal anatomic position.	
___	___	___	d. If using locking leather restraints, ensure that key is available at all times.	
___	___	___	e. Fasten restraint to the bed frame and not the side rail. Leather restraints come with leather straps that have buckles to secure to the bed frame. Site should not be readily accessible to the patient.	
___	___	___	6. Remove restraint at least every 2 hours or according to agency policy and patient need. When using leather restraints, care should be taken when releasing patient from restraint that harm does not come to the patient or the nurse. Consider releasing one extremity at a time.	
___	___	___	a. Check for signs of decreased circulation or impaired skin integrity.	
___	___	___	b. Perform range-of-motion exercises before re-applying.	
___	___	___	7. Reassure patient at regular intervals. Store call bell within easy reach.	

Excellent	Satisfactory	Needs Practice		Comments
			SKILL 3-4 **Applying Leather Restraints** *(Continued)*	
____	____	____	8. Assess for signs of sensory deprivation, such as increased sleeping, daydreaming, anxiety, panic, and hallucinations.	
____	____	____	9. Perform hand hygiene.	
____	____	____	10. Document reason for restraining patient, alternative measures attempted before applying the restraint, date and time of application, type of restraint, times when removed, and result and frequency of nursing assessment every 2 hours. Obtain a new order after 24 hours if restraints are still necessary.	

Skill Checklists to Accompany Taylor's Clinical Nursing Skills:
A Nursing Process Approach

Name _____   Date _____

Unit _____   Position _____

Instructor/Evaluator: _____   Position _____

SKILL 4-1

Hand Hygiene

Excellent	Satisfactory	Needs Practice		Comments

Goal: To maintain hands free of visible soiling.

1. Gather the necessary supplies. Stand in front of the sink. Do not allow your clothing to touch the sink during the washing procedure.
2. Remove jewelry, if possible, and secure in a safe place or allow plain wedding band to remain in place.
3. Turn on water and adjust force. Regulate the temperature until the water is warm.
4. Wet the hands and wrist area. Keep hands lower than elbows to allow water to flow toward fingertips.
5. Use about 1 teaspoon liquid soap from dispenser or rinse bar of soap and lather thoroughly. Cover all areas of hands with the soap product. Rinse soap bar again and return to soap dish.
6. With firm rubbing and circular motions, wash the palms and backs of the hands, each finger, the areas between the fingers, the knuckles, wrists, and forearms. Wash at least 1 inch above area of contamination. If hands are not visibly soiled, wash to 1 inch above the wrists.
7. Continue this friction motion for at least 15 seconds.
8. Use fingernails of the opposite hand or a clean orangewood stick to clean under fingernails.
9. Rinse thoroughly with water flowing toward fingertips.
10. Pat hands dry, beginning with the fingers and moving upward toward forearms, with a paper towel and discard it immediately. Use another clean towel to turn off the faucet. Discard towel immediately without touching other clean hand.
11. Use oil-free lotion on hands if desired.

Skill Checklists to Accompany Taylor's Clinical Nursing Skills:
A Nursing Process Approach

Name _____   Date _____

Unit _____   Position _____

Instructor/Evaluator: _____   Position _____

SKILL 4-2
Preparing a Sterile Field

Goal: To create a sterile field without evidence of contamination while keeping the patient free of exposure to potential infection causing microorganisms.

Excellent	Satisfactory	Needs Practice		Comments
___	___	___	1. Explain the procedure to the patient and perform hand hygiene.	
___	___	___	2. Check that sterile wrapped drape or package is dry and unopened. Also, note expiration date, making sure that the date is still valid.	
___	___	___	3. Select a work area that is waist level or higher.	
___	___	___	4. a. Open sterile wrapped drape or commercially prepared sterile package. For sterile wrapped drape, open outer covering. Remove sterile drape, lifting it carefully by its corners. Gently shake open, hold away from your body, and lay drape on selected work area.	
___	___	___	b. Place commercially prepared package in center of work area. Touching outer surface only, carefully reach around item and fold topmost flap of wrapper away from you. Open right and left flap before grasping the nearest flap and opening toward you.	
___	___	___	5. Place additional sterile items on field as needed.	
			When Adding a Sterile Item to a Sterile Field	
___	___	___	6. a. Hold agency wrapped item in one hand with top flap opening away from you. With other hand, unfold top flap and both sides. Keeping a secure hold on item, grasp the corners of the wrapper and pull back toward wrist, covering hand and wrist.	
___	___	___	b. If commercially packaged item has an unsealed corner, hold package in one hand and pull back on top cover with the other hand. If edge is partially sealed, use both hands to carefully peel apart.	
___	___	___	7. Drop sterile item onto sterile field from a 6-inch (15-cm) height or add item to field from the side. Be careful to avoid dropping onto 1-inch border.	
___	___	___	8. Discard wrapper.	

32

Excellent	Satisfactory	Needs Practice		Comments

SKILL 4-2
Preparing a Sterile Field *(Continued)*

When Pouring A Sterile Solution

— — — 9. Obtain appropriate solution and check expiration date.

— — — 10. Open solution container according to directions and place cap on table with edges up.

— — — 11. If bottle has previously been opened, "lip" it by pouring a small amount of solution into waste container.

— — — 12. Hold bottle outside the edge of the sterile field with the label side facing the palm of your hand and prepare to pour from a height of 4 to 6 inches (10 to 15 cm). The tip of the bottle should never touch a sterile container or dressing.

— — — 13. Pour required amount of solution steadily into sterile container positioned at side of sterile field. Avoid splashing any liquid.

— — — 14. Touch only the outside of the lid when recapping.

Copyright © 2005 by Lippincott Williams & Wilkins. *Skill Checklists to Accompany Taylor's Clinical Nursing Skills: A Nursing Process Approach,* by Pamela Evans-Smith and Marilee LeBon.

Skill Checklists to Accompany Taylor's Clinical Nursing Skills:
A Nursing Process Approach

Name _____   Date _____

Unit _____   Position _____

Instructor/Evaluator: _____   Position _____

Excellent	Satisfactory	Needs Practice	SKILL 4-3 **Donning and Removing Sterile Gloves**	
			Goal: To apply and remove gloves without contamination.	**Comments**
____	____	____	1. Perform hand hygiene.	
____	____	____	2. Place sterile glove package on clean dry surface at or above your waist.	
____	____	____	3. Open the outside wrapper by carefully peeling back top layer. Remove inner package, handling only the outside of it.	
____	____	____	4. Carefully open inner package using the flaps and expose sterile gloves with the cuff closest to you.	
____	____	____	5. With thumb and forefinger of nondominant hand, grasp folded cuff of sterile glove for dominant hand.	
____	____	____	6. Lift and hold glove up and off the inner package with fingers down. Be careful it does not touch any unsterile object.	
____	____	____	7. Carefully insert dominant hand palm up into glove and pull glove on.	
____	____	____	8. Holding thumb outward, slide fingers of gloved hand under cuff of remaining glove and lift glove upward.	
____	____	____	9. Carefully insert nondominant hand into glove. Adjust gloves on both hands, touching only sterile areas with other sterile areas.	
			To Remove Gloves	
____	____	____	10. Using dominant hand, grasp other glove near cuff end and remove by inverting it, keeping contaminated area on the inside. Continue to hold onto glove.	
____	____	____	11. Slide fingers of ungloved hand inside remaining glove. Grasp glove on inside and remove by turning inside out over hand and other glove.	
____	____	____	12. Discard gloves in appropriate container and perform hand hygiene.	

Skill Checklists to Accompany Taylor's Clinical Nursing Skills:
A Nursing Process Approach

Name _____ Date _____

Unit _____ Position _____

Instructor/Evaluator: _____ Position _____

Excellent	Satisfactory	Needs Practice	SKILL 4-4 **Using Personal Protection Equipment** **Goal:** To contain the transmission of microorganisms, keeping the patient free of exposure to potentially infectious microorganisms.	Comments
____	____	____	1. Check physician's order for type of precautions and review precautions in Infection Control Manual.	
____	____	____	2. Plan nursing activities and gather necessary equipment before entering patient's room.	
____	____	____	3. Provide instruction about precautions to patient, family members, and visitors.	
____	____	____	4. Perform hand hygiene.	
____	____	____	5. Put on gown, gloves, mask, and protective eyewear, if recommended, as precaution.	
____	____	____	a. Tie gown securely at neck and waist. Obtain waterproof gown if soiling is likely.	
____	____	____	b. Use clean disposable gloves. If worn with a gown, draw glove cuffs over gown sleeves.	
____	____	____	c. Securely tie and fit mask to face.	
____	____	____	d. Wear eyewear with face shields or protection on side of face.	
____	____	____	e. Alternatively, a combination of a mask and barrier device may be used.	
____	____	____	6. When patient care is completed, untie waist strings of gown, then remove gloves as follows:	
____	____	____	a. Grasp outside of one glove and turn inside out to remove.	
____	____	____	b. Insert fingers of ungloved hand inside cuff of remaining glove.	
____	____	____	c. Grasp glove and drop in appropriate container.	
____	____	____	7. After removing gloves, remove mask.	
			Surgical Mask	
____	____	____	a. Untie mask and drop by strings into waste container. For a mask with an elastic strap, lift strap from behind head and drop by strap into waste container.	

SKILL 4-4
Using Personal Protection Equipment (*Continued*)

Excellent	Satisfactory	Needs Practice		Comments
			Particulate Respirator	
___	___	___	a. Use hand to hold respirator in place.	
___	___	___	b. Pull bottom strap up and over head.	
___	___	___	c. Pull top strap over head.	
___	___	___	d. Remove respirator from face and save for future use (HEPA mask) or discard according to manufacturer's directions (disposable mask).	
___	___	___	8. Remove gown.	
			For Gown that Is Visibly Soiled	
___	___	___	a. Untie neck strings of gown. Remove gown without touching outside of gown by keeping one hand up and under gown cuff and using this protected hand to pull opposite sleeve down and off.	
___	___	___	b. Use ungowned arm and hand to grasp gown from the inside and remove from the remaining arm. Remove gown, turn inside out, and drop in appropriate container.	
___	___	___	9. Remove eyewear and clean according to agency policy.	
___	___	___	10. Perform hand hygiene.	

Skill Checklists to Accompany Taylor's Clinical Nursing Skills:
A Nursing Process Approach

Name _____ Date _____

Unit _____ Position _____

Instructor/Evaluator: _____ Position _____

Excellent	Satisfactory	Needs Practice	SKILL 5-1 **Administering Oral Medications**	Comments
			Goal: To provide a safe effective method of giving drugs intended for absorption in stomach and small intestine; the patient will swallow the medication without aspirating and will understand and comply with the medication regime.	
___	___	___	1. Gather equipment. Check each medication order against original physician's order according to agency policy. Clarify any inconsistencies. Check patient's chart for allergies.	
___	___	___	2. Know actions, special nursing considerations, safe dose ranges, purpose of administration, and adverse effects of medications to be administered.	
___	___	___	3. Perform hand hygiene.	
___	___	___	4. Move medication cart outside patient's room or prepare for administration in medication area.	
___	___	___	5. Unlock medication cart or drawer.	
___	___	___	6. Prepare medications for one patient at a time.	
___	___	___	7. Select the proper medication from drawer or stock and compare with Kardex or order. Check expiration dates and perform calculations if necessary.	
___	___	___	a. Place unit dose-packaged medications in a disposable cup. Do not open wrapper until at bedside. Keep narcotics and medications that require special nursing assessments in a separate container.	
___	___	___	b. When removing tablets or capsules from a bottle, pour the necessary number into bottle cap and then place tablets in a medication cup. Break only scored tablets, if necessary, to obtain proper dose. Do not touch tablets with hands.	
___	___	___	c. Hold liquid medication bottles with the label against palm. Use appropriate measuring device when pouring liquids and read the amount of medication at the bottom of the meniscus at eye level. Wipe bottle lip with a paper towel.	
___	___	___	8. Recheck each medication package or preparation with the order as it is poured.	
___	___	___	9. When all medications for one patient have been prepared, recheck once again with the medication order before taking them to patient.	

Administering Oral Medications *(Continued)*

Excellent	Satisfactory	Needs Practice		Comments
___	___	___	10. Carefully transport medications to patient's bedside. Keep medications in sight at all times.	
___	___	___	11. See that patient receives medications at the correct time.	
___	___	___	12. Identify the patient carefully. There are three correct ways to do this:	
___	___	___	a. Check name on patient's identification band.	
___	___	___	b. Ask patient to state his or her name.	
___	___	___	c. Verify patient's identification with a staff member who knows patient.	
___	___	___	13. Complete necessary assessments before administration of medications. Check allergy bracelet or ask patient about allergies. Explain purpose and action of each medication to patient.	
___	___	___	14. Assist patient to an upright or lateral position.	
___	___	___	15. Administer medications.	
___	___	___	a. Offer water or other permitted fluids with pills, capsules, tablets, and some liquid medications.	
___	___	___	b. Ask patient's preference regarding medications to be taken by hand or in a cup and one at a time or all at once.	
___	___	___	c. If capsule or tablet falls to the floor, discard it and administer a new one.	
___	___	___	d. Record any fluid intake if I-O measurement is ordered.	
___	___	___	16. Remain with patient until each medication is swallowed. Never leave medication at the patient's bedside. Unless you have seen patient swallow drug, you cannot record drug as having been administered.	
___	___	___	17. Perform hand hygiene.	
___	___	___	18. Record each medication given on medication chart or record using required format.	
___	___	___	a. If drug was refused or omitted, record this in appropriate area on medication record.	
___	___	___	b. Recording of administration of a narcotic may require additional documentation on a narcotic record stating drug count and other specific information.	
___	___	___	19. Check on patient within 30 minutes of drug administration to verify response to medication.	

Skill Checklists to Accompany Taylor's Clinical Nursing Skills:
A Nursing Process Approach

Name _____ Date _____

Unit _____ Position _____

Instructor/Evaluator: _____ Position _____

SKILL 5-2

Removing Medication from an Ampule

Goal: To safely withdraw prescribed drug dose from an ampule in a sterile manner free from glass shards.

Excellent	Satisfactory	Needs Practice		Comments
___	___	___	1. Gather equipment. Check medication order against original physician's order according to agency policy.	
___	___	___	2. Perform hand hygiene.	
___	___	___	3. Tap ampule stem or twist your wrist quickly while holding ampule vertically.	
___	___	___	4. Wrap a small gauze pad or dry antimicrobial swab around the neck of the ampule.	
___	___	___	5. Use a snapping motion to break off top of ampule along the prescored line at its neck. Always break away from your body.	
___	___	___	6. Remove the cap from the filter needle by pulling it straight off. Insert filter needle into ampule, being careful not to touch the rim.	
___	___	___	7. Withdraw medication in the amount ordered plus a small amount more (approximately 30%). Do not inject air into solutions. Use either of the following methods.	
___	___	___	a. Insert tip of needle into ampule, which is upright on a flat surface and withdraw fluid into syringe. Touch plunger at knob only.	
___	___	___	b. Insert tip of needle into ampule and invert ampule. Keep needle centered and not touching sides of ampule. Remove prescribed amount of medication. Touch plunger at knob only.	
___	___	___	8. Wait until needle has been withdrawn to tap syringe and expel air carefully. Do not expel any air bubbles that may form in the solution. Check amount of medication in syringe and discard any surplus.	
___	___	___	9. Discard ampule in a suitable container after comparing with medication Kardex.	
___	___	___	10. Discard the filter needle in a suitable container. If medication is to be given intramuscularly or if agency requires the use of a needle to administer medication, attach selected needle to syringe.	
___	___	___	11. Perform hand hygiene.	

Skill Checklists to Accompany Taylor's Clinical Nursing Skills:
A Nursing Process Approach

Name _____   Date _____

Unit _____   Position _____

Instructor/Evaluator: _____   Position _____

Excellent	Satisfactory	Needs Practice	SKILL 5-3 **Removing Medication from a Vial**	
			Goal: To safely withdraw prescribed drug dose from a vial in a sterile manner.	**Comments**
___ ___ ___			1. Gather equipment. Check medication order against original physician's order according to agency policy.	
___ ___ ___			2. Perform hand hygiene.	
___ ___ ___			3. Remove the metal or plastic cap on the vial that protects the rubber stopper.	
___ ___ ___			4. Swab rubber top with antimicrobial swab.	
___ ___ ___			5. Remove the cap from the needle by pulling it straight off. (Some agencies recommend use of a filter needle when withdrawing premixed medications from multidose vials.) Draw back an amount of air into syringe equal to specific dose of medication to be withdrawn.	
___ ___ ___			6. Pierce the rubber stopper in the center with the needle tip and inject measured air into the space above the solution. (Do not inject air into the solution.) Vial may be positioned upright on a flat surface or inverted.	
___ ___ ___			7. Invert vial and withdraw needle tip slightly so that it is below the fluid level.	
___ ___ ___			8. Draw up prescribed amount of medication while holding syringe at eye level and vertically. Be careful to touch the plunger at knob only.	
___ ___ ___			9. If any air bubbles accumulate in syringe, tap syringe barrel sharply and move needle past fluid into the air space to reinject the air bubble into vial. Return needle tip to the solution and continue withdrawal of medication.	
___ ___ ___			10. After correct dose is withdrawn, remove needle from vial and carefully replace cap over needle. If a filter needle has been used to draw up the medication and the medication needs to be administered through a needle, remove the filter needle and replace it with a new needle. (Some agencies recommend changing needles, if needed to administer the medication, before administering the medication.)	

Excellent	Satisfactory	Needs Practice	SKILL 5-3 **Removing Medication from a Vial** *(Continued)*	Comments
____	____	____	11. If using a multidose vial, label the vial with the date and time opened and store the vial containing remaining medication according to agency policy.	
____	____	____	12. Perform hand hygiene.	

Skill Checklists to Accompany Taylor's Clinical Nursing Skills:
A Nursing Process Approach

Name _____   Date _____

Unit _____   Position _____

Instructor/Evaluator: _____   Position _____

SKILL 5-4
Mixing Insulins in One Syringe

Goal: To safely withdraw prescribed insulin doses from two vials into one syringe with the insulin appropriately mixed in a sterile manner.

Excellent	Satisfactory	Needs Practice		Comments
___	___	___	1. Gather equipment. Check medication order against original physician's order according to agency policy.	
___	___	___	2. Perform hand hygiene.	
___	___	___	3. If necessary, remove cap that protects rubber stopper on each vial.	
___	___	___	4. If insulin is a suspension (NPH [neutral protamine Hagedorn], Lente), roll and agitate the vial to mix it well.	
___	___	___	5. Cleanse rubber tops with antimicrobial swabs.	
___	___	___	6. Remove cap from needle. Inject air into the modified insulin preparation (eg, NPH insulin). Touch plunger at knob only. Use an amount of air equal to the amount of medication to be withdrawn. Do not allow needle to touch medication in the vial. Remove needle.	
___	___	___	7. Inject air into the clear insulin without additional protein (eg, regular insulin). Use an amount of air equal to the amount of medication to be withdrawn.	
___	___	___	8. Invert the vial of clear insulin and aspirate the amount prescribed. Invert and then remove needle from vial.	
___	___	___	9. Cleanse rubber top of the modified insulin vial. Insert needle into this vial, invert it, and withdraw medication. Carefully replace cap over needle.	
___	___	___	10. Store vials according to agency recommendations.	
___	___	___	11. Perform hand hygiene.	

42

Skill Checklists to Accompany Taylor's Clinical Nursing Skills:
A Nursing Process Approach

Name _____ Date _____

Unit _____ Position _____

Instructor/Evaluator: _____ Position _____

Excellent	Satisfactory	Needs Practice	SKILL 5-5 **Administering an Intradermal Injection**	Comments
			Goal: To safely deliver prescribed drug dose to area just below the epidermis, producing the appearance of a wheal or blister at the site of injection.	
___	___	___	1. Assemble equipment and check physician's order.	
___	___	___	2. Explain procedure to patient.	
___	___	___	3. Perform hand hygiene. Don disposable gloves.	
___	___	___	4. If necessary, withdraw medication from ampule or vial as described in Skills 5-2 and 5-3, respectively.	
___	___	___	5. Select area on inner aspect of forearm that is not heavily pigmented or covered with hair. Upper chest or upper back beneath the scapulae are also sites for intradermal injections.	
___	___	___	6. Cleanse the area with an antimicrobial swab by wiping with a firm circular motion and moving outward from the injection site. Allow skin to dry. If skin is oily, clean area with pledget moistened with acetone.	
___	___	___	7. Use nondominant hand to spread skin taut over injection site.	
___	___	___	8. Remove needle cap with nondominant hand by pulling it straight off.	
___	___	___	9. Place needle almost flat against patient's skin, bevel side up. Insert needle into skin so that point of the needle can be seen through skin. Insert needle only about ⅛ inch with the entire bevel under the skin.	
___	___	___	10. Slowly inject agent while watching for a small wheal or blister to appear. If none appears, withdraw needle to ensure bevel is in interdermal tissue.	
___	___	___	11. Once the agent has been injected, withdraw needle quickly at the same angle it was inserted.	
___	___	___	12. Do not massage area after removing needle. Tell the patient not to rub or scratch the site.	
___	___	___	13. Do not recap used needle. Discard needle and syringe in the appropriate receptacle.	
___	___	___	14. Assist patient into a position of comfort.	
___	___	___	15. Remove gloves and dispose of them properly. Perform hand hygiene.	

Excellent	Satisfactory	Needs Practice	SKILL 5-5 **Administering an Intradermal Injection** *(Continued)*	
				Comments
——	——	——	16. Chart administration of medication and site of administration. Charting may be documented on computerized medication administration record (CMAR), including location.	
——	——	——	17. Observe the area for signs of a reaction at ordered intervals, usually at 24- to 72-hour periods. Inform the patient of this inspection.	

Skill Checklists to Accompany Taylor's Clinical Nursing Skills:
A Nursing Process Approach

Name _____   Date _____

Unit _____   Position _____

Instructor/Evaluator: _____   Position _____

SKILL 5-6
Administering a Subcutaneous Injection

Goal: To safely deliver prescribed drug dose into subcutaneous tissue.

Excellent	Satisfactory	Needs Practice		Comments
___	___	___	1. Assemble equipment and check physician's order.	
___	___	___	2. Explain procedure to patient.	
___	___	___	3. Perform hand hygiene.	
___	___	___	4. If necessary, withdraw medication from ampule or vial as described in Skills 5-2 and 5-3, respectively.	
___	___	___	5. Identify patient carefully by checking the identification band on the patient's wrist and asking the patient his or her name. Close curtain to provide privacy. Don disposable gloves.	
___	___	___	6. Have patient assume a position appropriate for the most commonly used sites:	
___	___	___	a. Outer aspect of upper arm—Patient's arm should be relaxed and at side of body.	
___	___	___	b. Anterior thighs—Patient may sit or lie with leg relaxed.	
___	___	___	c. Abdomen—Patient may lie in a semirecumbent position.	
___	___	___	7. Locate site of choice according to directions given in Box 5-5 of *Taylor's Clinical Nursing Skills.* Ensure that area is not tender and is free of lumps or nodules.	
___	___	___	8. Clean area around injection site with an antimicrobial swab. Use a firm circular motion while moving outward from the injection site. Allow area to dry.	
___	___	___	9. Remove needle cap with nondominant hand, pulling it straight off.	
___	___	___	10. Grasp and bunch area surrounding injection site or spread skin at site.	
___	___	___	11. Hold syringe in dominant hand between thumb and forefinger. Inject needle quickly at an angle of 45 to 90 degrees, depending on amount and turgor of tissue and length of needle.	
___	___	___	12. After needle is in place, release tissue. If you have a large skin fold pinched up, ensure that the needle stays in place as the skin is released. Immediately move your	

Administering a Subcutaneous Injection *(Continued)*

Excellent	Satisfactory	Needs Practice		Comments
			nondominant hand to steady the lower end of the syringe. Slide your dominant hand to the tip of the barrel.	
____	____	____	13. Aspirate, if recommended, by pulling back gently on syringe plunger to determine whether needle is in a blood vessel. If blood appears, the needle should be withdrawn, the medication syringe and needle discarded, and a new syringe with medication prepared. Do not aspirate when giving insulin or heparin.	
____	____	____	14. If no blood appears, inject solution slowly.	
____	____	____	15. Withdraw needle quickly at the same angle at which it was inserted.	
____	____	____	16. Massage area gently with cotton ball or dry swab. (Do not massage a subcutaneous heparin or insulin injection site.) Apply a small bandage if needed.	
____	____	____	17. Do not recap used needle. Discard needle and syringe in appropriate receptacle.	
____	____	____	18. Assist patient to a position of comfort.	
____	____	____	19. Remove gloves, and dispose of them properly. Perform hand hygiene.	
____	____	____	20. Chart administration of medication, including the site of administration. This charting can be done on CMAR.	
____	____	____	21. Evaluate patient response to medication within an appropriate time frame.	

Skill Checklists to Accompany Taylor's Clinical Nursing Skills:
A Nursing Process Approach

Name _____ Date _____

Unit _____ Position _____

Instructor/Evaluator: _____ Position _____

Excellent	Satisfactory	Needs Practice	SKILL 5-7 **Administering an Intramuscular Injection**	
			Goal: To safely deliver prescribed drug dose into muscle tissue.	**Comments**
____	____	____	1. Assemble equipment and check physician's order.	
____	____	____	2. Explain procedure to patient.	
____	____	____	3. Perform hand hygiene.	
____	____	____	4. If necessary, withdraw medication from ampule or vial as described in Skills 5-2 and 5-3, respectively.	
____	____	____	5. Do not add air to syringe.	
____	____	____	6. Identify the patient carefully. There are three ways to do this:	
____	____	____	a. Check the name on the patient's identification badge.	
____	____	____	b. Ask the patient his or her name.	
____	____	____	c. Verify the patient's identification with a staff member who knows the patient.	
____	____	____	7. Provide for privacy. Have patient assume a position for the site selected:	
____	____	____	a. Ventrogluteal—Patient may lie on back or side with hip and knee flexed.	
____	____	____	b. Vastus lateralis—Patient may lie on the back or may assume a sitting position.	
____	____	____	c. Deltoid—Patient may sit or lie with arm relaxed.	
____	____	____	d. Dorsogluteal—Patient may lie prone with toes pointing inward or on side with upper leg flexed and placed in front of lower leg.	
____	____	____	8. Locate site of choice according to directions given in Box 5-6 of *Taylor's Clinical Nursing Skills*. Ensure that the area is not tender and is free of lumps or nodules. Don disposable gloves.	
____	____	____	9. Clean area thoroughly with antimicrobial swab, using friction. Allow alcohol to dry.	
____	____	____	10. Remove needle cap by pulling it straight off.	
____	____	____	11. Displace skin in a Z-track manner by pulling to one side, or spread skin at the site using your nondominant hand.	

Excellent	Satisfactory	Needs Practice		

SKILL 5-7
Administering an Intramuscular Injection *(Continued)*

Comments

Excellent	Satisfactory	Needs Practice		
⎯⎯	⎯⎯	⎯⎯	12. Hold syringe in your dominant hand between thumb and forefinger. Quickly dart needle into the tissue at a 90-degree angle.	
⎯⎯	⎯⎯	⎯⎯	13. As soon as needle is in place, move your nondominant hand to hold lower end of syringe. Slide your dominant hand to tip of barrel.	
⎯⎯	⎯⎯	⎯⎯	14. Aspirate by slowly (for at least 5 seconds) pulling back on plunger to determine whether the needle is in a blood vessel. If blood is aspirated, discard needle, syringe, and medication. Prepare a new sterile setup and inject in another site.	
⎯⎯	⎯⎯	⎯⎯	15. If no blood is aspirated, inject solution slowly (10 seconds/mL of medication).	
⎯⎯	⎯⎯	⎯⎯	16. Remove needle slowly and steadily. Release displaced tissue if Z-track technique was used.	
⎯⎯	⎯⎯	⎯⎯	17. Apply gentle pressure at site with a small dry sponge.	
⎯⎯	⎯⎯	⎯⎯	18. Do not recap used needle. Discard needle and syringe in appropriate receptacle.	
⎯⎯	⎯⎯	⎯⎯	19. Assist patient to a position of comfort. Encourage patient to exercise extremity used for injection if possible.	
⎯⎯	⎯⎯	⎯⎯	20. Remove gloves and dispose of them properly. Perform hand hygiene.	
⎯⎯	⎯⎯	⎯⎯	21. Chart administration of medication including the site of administration. This may be documented on the CMAR.	
⎯⎯	⎯⎯	⎯⎯	22. Evaluate patient response to medication within an appropriate time frame. Assess site, if possible, within 2 to 4 hours after administration.	

Skill Checklists to Accompany Taylor's Clinical Nursing Skills:
A Nursing Process Approach

Name _____ Date _____

Unit _____ Position _____

Instructor/Evaluator: _____ Position _____

Excellent	Satisfactory	Needs Practice	SKILL 5-8 **Adding Medications to an Intravenous Solution**	Comments
			Goal: To safely introduce prescribed drug dose into an intravenous solution and mix appropriately.	
___	___	___	1. Gather all equipment and bring to patient's bedside. Check medication order against physician's order, and that medication is compatible with IV fluid. Take the equipment to patient's bedside.	
___	___	___	2. Perform hand hygiene.	
___	___	___	3. Identify patient by checking the band on the patient's wrist and asking patient his or her name. Check for any allergies the patient may have.	
___	___	___	4. Explain the procedure to the patient.	
___	___	___	5. Add medications to intravenous (IV) solution that is infusing.	
___	___	___	a. Check that volume in bag or bottle is adequate.	
___	___	___	b. Close IV clamp.	
___	___	___	c. Clean medication port with antimicrobial swab.	
___	___	___	d. Steady container. Uncap needle or needleless device and insert it into port. Inject medication.	
___	___	___	e. Remove container from IV pole and gently rotate solution.	
___	___	___	f. Rehang container, open clamp, and readjust flow rate.	
___	___	___	g. Attach label to container so that dose of added medication is apparent.	
___	___	___	6. Add medication to IV solution before infusion.	
___	___	___	a. Carefully remove any protective cover and locate injection port. Clean with antimicrobial swab.	
___	___	___	b. Uncap needle or needleless device and insert into port. Inject medication.	
___	___	___	c. Withdraw needle and insert spike into proper entry site on bag or bottle.	
___	___	___	d. With tubing clamped, gently rotate IV solution in the bag or bottle. Hang the IV bag.	
___	___	___	e. Attach the label to the container so that dose of added medication is apparent.	

Excellent	Satisfactory	Needs Practice		
			SKILL 5-8 **Adding Medications to an Intravenous Solution** (*Continued*)	
				Comments
——	——	——	7. Dispose of equipment according to agency policy.	
——	——	——	8. Perform hand hygiene.	
——	——	——	9. Chart addition of medication to IV solution. This may be done on the CMAR.	
——	——	——	10. Evaluate patient's response to medication within appropriate time frame.	

50

Name _____   Date _____

Unit _____   Position _____

Instructor/Evaluator: _____   Position _____

Excellent	Satisfactory	Needs Practice	SKILL 5-9 **Adding a Bolus Intravenous Medication to an Existing Intravenous Line**	
			Goal: To safely introduce prescribed drug dose directly into intravenous line.	**Comments**
___	___	___	1. Gather equipment and bring to patient's bedside. Check medication order against physician's order. Check a drug resource to clarify if medication needs to be diluted before administration.	
___	___	___	2. Explain procedure to patient.	
___	___	___	3. Perform hand hygiene. Don clean gloves.	
___	___	___	4. Identify patient by checking the band on the patient's wrist and asking patient his or her name.	
___	___	___	5. Assess IV site for presence of inflammation or infiltration.	
___	___	___	6. Select the injection port on tubing closest to the venipuncture site. Clean port with antimicrobial swab.	
___	___	___	7. Uncap syringe. Steady port with your nondominant hand while inserting needleless device or needle into the center of port.	
___	___	___	8. Move your nondominant hand to the section of IV tubing directly behind or just distal to injection port. Fold the tubing between your fingers to temporarily stop the flow of IV solution.	
___	___	___	9. Pull back slightly on plunger just until blood appears in tubing. If no blood appears, medication may still be administered while assessing IV insertion site for signs of infiltration.	
___	___	___	10. Inject medication at the recommended rate.	
___	___	___	11. Remove needle. Do not cap it. Release tubing and allow IV to flow at the proper rate.	
___	___	___	12. Dispose of syringe in proper receptacle.	
___	___	___	13. Remove gloves and perform hand hygiene.	
___	___	___	14. Chart administration of medication. This may be done on the CMAR.	
___	___	___	15. Evaluate patient's response to medication within appropriate time frame.	

Skill Checklists to Accompany Taylor's Clinical Nursing Skills:
A Nursing Process Approach

Name _____   Date _____

Unit _____   Position _____

Instructor/Evaluator: _____   Position _____

Excellent	Satisfactory	Needs Practice	SKILL 5-10 **Administering Intravenous Medications by Piggyback, Volume Control Administration Set, or Mini-Infusion Pump** **Goal:** To safely deliver prescribed drug dose by intravenous infusion over a short period at the prescribed interval.	Comments
____	____	____	1. Gather all equipment and bring to patient's bedside. Check medication order against original physician's order according to agency policy.	
____	____	____	2. Identify patient by checking the identification band on patient's wrist and asking patient his or her name.	
____	____	____	3. Explain procedure to patient.	
____	____	____	4. Perform hand hygiene and don gloves.	
____	____	____	5. Assess IV site for presence of inflammation or infiltration.	
			Using Piggyback Infusion	
____	____	____	6. Attach infusion tubing to the piggyback set containing diluted medication. Place label on tubing with appropriate date and attach needle or needleless device to end of tubing according to manufacturer's directions. Open clamp and prime tubing. Close clamp.	
____	____	____	7. Hang piggyback container on IV pole, positioning it higher than the primary IV bag according to manufacturer's recommendations. Use metal or plastic hook to lower primary IV bag.	
____	____	____	8. Use antimicrobial swab to clean appropriate port.	
____	____	____	9. Connect piggyback setup to either	
____	____	____	a. Needleless port;	
____	____	____	b. Stopcock: Turn stopcock to open position;	
____	____	____	c. Primary IV line: Uncap needle and insert into secondary IV port closest to the top of the primary tubing. Use a strip of tape to secure secondary set tubing to primary infusion tubing. Primary line is left unclamped if port has a back-flow valve.	
____	____	____	10. Open clamp on piggyback set and regulate flow at the prescribed delivery rate or set rate for secondary infusion on infusion pump. Monitor medication infusion at periodic intervals.	

Excellent	Satisfactory	Needs Practice	SKILL 5-10 **Administering Intravenous Medications by Piggyback, Volume Control Administration Set, or Mini-Infusion Pump** (*Continued*)
			Comments
―	―	―	11. Clamp tubing on piggyback set when solution is infused. Follow agency policy regarding disposal of equipment.
―	―	―	12. Readjust flow rate of the primary IV line.
			Using a Mini-Infusion Pump
―	―	―	13. Connect prepared syringe to mini-infusion tubing.
―	―	―	14. Fill tubing with medication by applying gentle pressure to syringe plunger.
―	―	―	15. Insert syringe into mini-infuser pump as per manufacturer's directions.
―	―	―	16. Use an antimicrobial swab to cleanse the appropriate connector. Connect mini-infusion tubing to appropriate connector as in Action 9.
―	―	―	17. Program pump to begin infusion. Set alarm if recommended by manufacturer.
―	―	―	18. Recheck flow rate of primary IV line once pump has completed delivery of medication.
			Using a Volume Control Administration Set
―	―	―	19. Withdraw medication from ampule or vial into prepared syringe as described in Skills 5-2 and 5-3, respectively.
―	―	―	20. Open clamp between IV solution and the volume control administration set or secondary setup. Follow manufacturer's instructions and fill with desired amount of IV solution. Close clamp.
―	―	―	21. Use an antimicrobial swab to clean injection port on the secondary setup.
―	―	―	22. Remove clamp and insert needle or blunt needleless device into port while holding syringe steady. Inject medication. Mix gently with IV solution.
―	―	―	23. Open clamp below the secondary setup and regulate at prescribed delivery rate. Monitor medication infusion at periodic intervals.
―	―	―	24. Attach medication label to volume control device.
―	―	―	25. Place syringe with uncapped needle in designated container.
―	―	―	26. Perform hand hygiene.
―	―	―	27. Chart administration of medication after it has been infused. This can be done on the CMAR.
―	―	―	28. Evaluate patient's response to medication within appropriate time frame.

Skill Checklists to Accompany Taylor's Clinical Nursing Skills:
A Nursing Process Approach

Name _____ Date _____

Unit _____ Position _____

Instructor/Evaluator: _____ Position _____

SKILL 5-11
Introducing Drugs through a Heparin or Intravenous Lock Using Saline Flush

Goal: To safely deliver prescribed drug dose by intravenous infusion over a short period at the prescribed interval into a heparin or intravenous lock device.

Excellent	Satisfactory	Needs Practice		Comments
___	___	___	1. Assemble equipment and check physician's order.	
___	___	___	2. Identify the person by checking the identification band on the patient's wrist and asking the patient his or her name. Explain the procedure to the patient.	
___	___	___	3. Perform hand hygiene.	
___	___	___	4. Withdraw 1 to 2 mL of sterile saline from vial into syringe as described in Skill 5-3.	
___	___	___	5. Don clean gloves and prepare to administer medication.	
___	___	___	6. Administer medication.	
			For Bolus Intravenous Injection	
___	___	___	a. Check drug package for correct injection rate for the IV push route.	
___	___	___	b. Clean port of the lock with antimicrobial swab.	
___	___	___	c. Stabilize port with your nondominant hand and insert needleless device or needle of syringe of normal saline into the port.	
___	___	___	d. Aspirate gently and check for blood return. (Blood return does not always occur even though lock is patent.)	
___	___	___	e. Gently flush with 1 mL of normal saline. Remove syringe.	
___	___	___	f. Insert blunt needleless device or needle of syringe with medication into port and gently inject medication, using a watch to verify correct injection rate. Do not force the injection if there is resistance. If lock is clogged, it has to be changed. Remove medication syringe and needle when administration is completed.	
___	___	___	g. Remove syringe with medication from port. Stabilize the port with your nondominant hand and insert the needleless device or needle of syringe of normal saline into the port. Slowly flush the reservoir with 1 to 2 mL of sterile saline using positive pressure. To gain positive	

Excellent	Satisfactory	Needs Practice	SKILL 5-11 **Introducing Drugs through a Heparin or Intravenous Lock Using Saline Flush** *(Continued)*	Comments
			pressure, you can either clamp the IV tubing as you are still flushing the last of the saline into the IV line or remove the syringe as you are still flushing the remainder of the saline into the IV line. Remove the syringe and discard uncapped needles and syringes in the appropriate receptacle. Remove gloves and discard appropriately.	
			For Administration of a Drug by Way of an Intermittent Delivery System	
——	——	——	7. a. Use a drug resource book to check correct flow rate of medication. (Usual rate is 30 to 60 minutes).	
——	——	——	b. Connect infusion tubing to the medication setup according to manufacturer's directions using sterile technique. Hang IV setup on a pole. Open clamp and allow solution to clear IV tubing of air. Reclamp tubing.	
——	——	——	c. Attach needleless connector or sterile 25-gauge needle to end of infusion tubing.	
——	——	——	d. Clean port of the lock with antimicrobial swab.	
——	——	——	e. Stabilize port with your nondominant hand and insert needleless device or needle of syringe of normal saline into the port.	
——	——	——	f. Aspirate gently and check for blood return. (Blood return does not always occur even though lock is patent.)	
——	——	——	g. Gently flush with 1 mL of normal saline. Remove syringe.	
——	——	——	h. Insert blunt needleless device or needle attached to tubing into port. If necessary, secure with tape.	
——	——	——	i. Open clamp and regulate flow rate or attach to IV pump or controller according to manufacturer's directions. Close clamp when infusion is complete.	
——	——	——	j. Remove the needleless connector or needle from lock. Carefully replace uncapped used needle or needleless device with a new sterile one. Allow medication setup to hang on the pole for future use according to agency policy. Stabilize port with your nondominant hand and insert needleless device or needle of syringe of normal saline into the port. Slowly flush the reservoir with 1 to 2 mL of sterile saline using positive pressure. To gain positive pressure, you can either clamp the IV tubing as	

SKILL 5-11
Introducing Drugs through a Heparin or Intravenous Lock Using Saline Flush *(Continued)*

Excellent	Satisfactory	Needs Practice		Comments
			you are still flushing the last of the saline into the IV or remove the syringe as you are still flushing the remainder of the saline into the IV line. Remove syringe and discard uncapped needles and syringes in appropriate receptacle. Remove gloves and discard appropriately.	
___	___	___	8. Perform hand hygiene.	
___	___	___	9. Check the injection site and IV lock at least every 8 hours and administer a small amount of saline (2 to 3 mL) if medication is not given at least every 8 to 12 hours.	
___	___	___	10. Change the heparin lock at least every 72 to 96 hours or according to agency policy. A lock that is not patent should be changed immediately.	
___	___	___	11. Chart the administration of the medication or saline flush.	

Skill Checklists to Accompany Taylor's Clinical Nursing Skills:
A Nursing Process Approach

Name _____ Date _____

Unit _____ Position _____

Instructor/Evaluator: _____ Position _____

SKILL 5-12

Applying a Transdermal Patch

Goal: To successfully deliver medication via the transdermal route.

Excellent	Satisfactory	Needs Practice		Comments
___	___	___	1. Bring equipment to patient's bedside. Check the medication order against the original physician's order according to agency policy.	
___	___	___	2. Identify the person by checking the identification band on the patient's wrist and asking the patient his or her name. Ask patient about any allergies.	
___	___	___	3. Explain the procedure to the patient.	
___	___	___	4. Perform hand hygiene and don gloves.	
___	___	___	5. Assess the patient's skin where patch is to be placed, looking for any signs of irritation or any areas that are broken down. Find place that does not have a large amount of hair. If patient has a large amount of hair on chest or back, scissors may be used to trim hair. Do not shave hair.	
___	___	___	6. Remove any old transdermal patches that are left on patient. Gently wash the area where the old patch was with soap and water.	
___	___	___	7. Remove cover without touching the adhesive side. Lie patch on patient's skin, pressing firmly with palm of hand for 10 seconds.	
___	___	___	8. On transdermal patch, write your initials, date, and time.	
___	___	___	9. Remove gloves and perform hand hygiene.	
___	___	___	10. Chart the site of administration of medication after the patch has been placed. This may be done on the CMAR.	
___	___	___	11. Evaluate the patient's response to medication within the appropriate time frame.	

Skill Checklists to Accompany Taylor's Clinical Nursing Skills:
A Nursing Process Approach

Name _____   Date _____

Unit _____   Position _____

Instructor/Evaluator: _____   Position _____

SKILL 5-13

Instilling Eyedrops

Excellent	Satisfactory	Needs Practice	**Goal:** To successfully deliver medication to the eye.	Comments
___	___	___	1. Bring equipment to patient's bedside. Check the medication order against the original physician's order according to agency policy.	
___	___	___	2. Identify the person by checking the identification band on the patient's wrist and asking the patient his or her name. Ask the patient about any allergies.	
___	___	___	3. Explain the procedure to the patient.	
___	___	___	4. Perform hand hygiene and don gloves.	
___	___	___	5. Offer tissue to patient.	
___	___	___	6. Cleanse the eyelids and eyelashes of any drainage with a washcloth moistened with normal saline solution proceeding from the inner canthus to the outer canthus. Use each area of the washcloth only once.	
___	___	___	7. Tilt the patient's head back slightly. The head may be turned slightly to the affected side.	
___	___	___	8. Remove the cap from the medication bottle, being careful to not touch the inner side of the cap.	
___	___	___	9. Invert the monodrip plastic container that is commonly used to instill eyedrops. Have the patient look up while focusing on something on the ceiling.	
___	___	___	10. Place the thumb or two fingers near the margin of the lower eyelid immediately below the eyelashes and exert pressure downward over the bony prominence of the cheek. The lower conjunctival sac is exposed as the lower lid is pulled down.	
___	___	___	11. Hold the dropper close to the eye, but avoid touching the eyelids or lashes. Squeeze the container and allow the prescribed number of drops to fall in the lower conjunctival sac.	
___	___	___	12. Release the lower lid after the eyedrops are instilled. Ask the patient to close the eyes gently.	
___	___	___	13. Apply gentle pressure over the inner canthus to prevent the eyedrops from flowing into the tear duct.	

58

Excellent	Satisfactory	Needs Practice	SKILL 5-13 **Instilling Eyedrops** *(Continued)*	
				Comments
___	___	___	14. Instruct patient not to rub affected eye.	
___	___	___	15. Remove gloves and perform hand hygiene.	
___	___	___	16. Chart the administration of medication after the drops have been administered. This may be done on the CMAR.	
___	___	___	17. Evaluate the patient's response to medication within the appropriate time frame.	

Skill Checklists to Accompany Taylor's Clinical Nursing Skills:
A Nursing Process Approach

Name _____   Date _____

Unit _____   Position _____

Instructor/Evaluator: _____   Position _____

Excellent	Satisfactory	Needs Practice	SKILL 5-14 **Administering an Eye Irrigation**	Comments
			Goal: To successfully cleanse the eye of a patient.	
⎯⎯	⎯⎯	⎯⎯	1. Explain procedure to patient.	
⎯⎯	⎯⎯	⎯⎯	2. Assemble equipment at patient's bedside.	
⎯⎯	⎯⎯	⎯⎯	3. Perform hand hygiene.	
⎯⎯	⎯⎯	⎯⎯	4. Have the patient sit or lie with the head tilted toward the side of the affected eye. Protect the patient and the bed with a waterproof pad.	
⎯⎯	⎯⎯	⎯⎯	5. Don disposable gloves. Clean the lids and the lashes with a washcloth moistened with normal saline or the solution ordered for the irrigation. Wipe from the inner canthus to outer canthus. Use a different corner of washcloth with each wipe.	
⎯⎯	⎯⎯	⎯⎯	6. Place the curved basin at the cheek on the side of the affected eye to receive the irrigating solution. If the patient is sitting up, ask him or her to support the basin.	
⎯⎯	⎯⎯	⎯⎯	7. Expose the lower conjunctival sac and hold the upper lid open with your nondominant hand.	
⎯⎯	⎯⎯	⎯⎯	8. Hold the irrigator about 2.5 cm (1 inch) from the eye. Direct the flow of the solution from the inner to the outer canthus along the conjunctival sac.	
⎯⎯	⎯⎯	⎯⎯	9. Irrigate until the solution is clear or all the solution has been used. Use only sufficient force to remove secretions gently from the conjunctiva. Avoid touching any part of the eye with the irrigating tip.	
⎯⎯	⎯⎯	⎯⎯	10. Have the patient close the eye periodically during the procedure.	
⎯⎯	⎯⎯	⎯⎯	11. Dry the area after the irrigation with a gauze sponge. Offer a towel to the patient if the face and neck are wet.	
⎯⎯	⎯⎯	⎯⎯	12. Remove gloves and perform hand hygiene.	
⎯⎯	⎯⎯	⎯⎯	13. Chart the irrigation, appearance of the eye, drainage, and the patient's response.	

Skill Checklists to Accompany Taylor's Clinical Nursing Skills:
A Nursing Process Approach

Name _____ Date _____

Unit _____ Position _____

Instructor/Evaluator: _____ Position _____

SKILL 5-15
Instilling Eardrops

Goal: To successfully administer eardrops to a patient.

Excellent	Satisfactory	Needs Practice		Comments
___	___	___	1. Bring equipment to patient's bedside. Check physician's order.	
___	___	___	2. Identify the person by checking the identification band on the patient's wrist and asking the patient his or her name. Ask patient regarding any medication allergies.	
___	___	___	3. Explain the procedure to the patient.	
___	___	___	4. Perform hand hygiene and don gloves (gloves are to be worn if drainage is present).	
___	___	___	5. Offer tissue to patient.	
___	___	___	6. Cleanse the external ear of any drainage with a cotton ball or a washcloth moistened with normal saline.	
___	___	___	7. Place the patient on the unaffected side in bed or, if ambulatory, have the patient sit with the head well tilted to the side so that the affected ear is uppermost.	
___	___	___	8. Draw up the amount of solution needed in the dropper. Excess medication should not be returned to a stock bottle. A prepackaged monodrip plastic container may also be used.	
___	___	___	9. Straighten the auditory canal by pulling the cartilaginous portion of the pinna up and back in an adult and down and back in an infant or a child under the age of 3 years.	
___	___	___	10. Hold the dropper in the ear with its tip above the auditory canal. For an infant or an irrational or confused patient, protect the dropper with a piece of soft tubing to help prevent injury to the ear.	
___	___	___	11. Allow the drops to fall on the side of the canal.	
___	___	___	12. Release the pinna after instilling the drops and have the patient maintain the position to prevent the escape of medication.	
___	___	___	13. Gently press on the tragus a few times.	
___	___	___	14. If ordered, loosely insert a cotton ball into ear canal.	
___	___	___	15. Remove gloves and perform hand hygiene.	

Instilling Eardrops *(Continued)*

Excellent	Satisfactory	Needs Practice		Comments
___	___	___	16. Document the medication administration and any drainage from the ear noted. The medication documentation may be done on CMAR.	

Name _____ Date _____

Unit _____ Position _____

Instructor/Evaluator: _____ Position _____

Excellent	Satisfactory	Needs Practice	SKILL 5-16 **Administering an Ear Irrigation**	
			Goal: To safely cleanse external auditory canal.	**Comments**
___	___	___	1. Explain procedure to patient.	
___	___	___	2. Bring equipment to patient's bedside. Check physician's order. Protect patient and bed linens with a moisture-proof pad.	
___	___	___	3. Perform hand hygiene.	
___	___	___	4. Have patient sit up or lie with head tilted toward the side of the affected ear. Have patient support a basin under the ear to receive the irrigating solution.	
___	___	___	5. Clean pinna and meatus at the auditory canal as necessary with applicators dipped in warm tap water or irrigating solution.	
___	___	___	6. Fill bulb syringe with solution. If using an irrigating container, allow air to escape from tubing.	
___	___	___	7. Straighten auditory canal by pulling the pinna up and back for an adult, straight and back for a child over 3 years of age, and down and back for an infant or child up to 3 years of age.	
___	___	___	8. Direct a steady slow stream of solution against roof of auditory canal, using only sufficient force to remove secretions. Do not occlude auditory canal with irrigating nozzle. Allow solution to flow out unimpeded.	
___	___	___	9. When irrigation solution is completed, place cotton ball loosely in the auditory meatus and have patient lie on the side of the affected ear on a towel or absorbent pad.	
___	___	___	10. Perform hand hygiene.	
___	___	___	11. Chart irrigation, appearance of drainage, and patient's response.	
___	___	___	12. Return in 10 to 15 minutes and remove cotton ball and assess drainage.	

Skill Checklists to Accompany Taylor's Clinical Nursing Skills:
A Nursing Process Approach

Name _____   Date _____

Unit _____   Position _____

Instructor/Evaluator: _____   Position _____

SKILL 5-17

Instilling Nose Drops

Goal: To successfully administer medication in the form of nose drops.

Excellent	Satisfactory	Needs Practice		Comments
____	____	____	1. Bring equipment to patient's bedside. Check physician's order.	
____	____	____	2. Identify the person by checking the identification band on the patient's wrist and asking the patient his or her name. Also ask patient about any medication allergies.	
____	____	____	3. Explain the procedure to the patient.	
____	____	____	4. Perform hand hygiene and don gloves (gloves are to be worn if drainage is present).	
____	____	____	5. Provide the patient with paper tissues and ask patient to blow his or her nose.	
____	____	____	6. Have the patient sit up with head tilted well back. Or, if the patient is lying down, tilt the head back over a pillow.	
____	____	____	7. Draw sufficient solution into the dropper for both nares. Excess solution should not be returned to a stock bottle.	
____	____	____	8. Hold up the tip of the nose and place the dropper just inside the nares about one-third of an inch. Instill the prescribed number of drops in one naris and then into the other. Protect the dropper with a piece of soft tubing when the patient is an infant or young child. Avoid touching the nares with the dropper.	
____	____	____	9. Have the patient remain in position with the head tilted back for a few minutes.	
____	____	____	10. Document the medication administration and any drainage from nose noted. The medication documentation may be done on the CMAR.	

Skill Checklists to Accompany Taylor's Clinical Nursing Skills:
A Nursing Process Approach

Name _____   Date _____

Unit _____   Position _____

Instructor/Evaluator: _____   Position _____

Excellent	Satisfactory	Needs Practice	SKILL 5-18 **Inserting a Vaginal Suppository or Cream**	Comments
			Goal: To successfully administer medication in the form of a vaginal suppository or cream.	
___	___	___	1. Bring equipment to patient's bedside. Check physician's order.	
___	___	___	2. Identify the person by checking the identification band on the patient's wrist and asking the patient her name. Ask the patient about any medication allergies.	
___	___	___	3. Explain the procedure to the patient. Provide privacy.	
___	___	___	4. Perform hand hygiene and don gloves.	
___	___	___	5. Fill a vaginal applicator with the prescribed amount of cream or have a suppository ready.	
___	___	___	6. Lubricate the applicator with water, as necessary. A suppository may be lubricated with a water-soluble gel.	
___	___	___	7. Spread the labia well with the fingers and clean the area at the vaginal orifice with a washcloth and warm water, using a different corner of the washcloth with each stroke. Wipe from above the orifice downward toward the sacrum (front to back).	
			Administering a Vaginal Cream with Applicator	
___	___	___	8. Introduce the applicator gently in a rolling manner while directing it downward and backward.	
___	___	___	9. After the applicator is properly positioned, the labia may be allowed to fall in place if necessary to free the hand for manipulating the plunger. Push the plunger to its full length and then gently remove the applicator with the plunger depressed.	
			Inserting a Vaginal Suppository	
___	___	___	10. Insert suppository well into the vagina.	
___	___	___	11. Ask the patient to remain in the supine position for 5 to 10 minutes after the insertion.	
___	___	___	12. Offer the patient a perineal pad to collect excess drainage.	
___	___	___	13. Remove gloves and perform hand hygiene.	
___	___	___	14. Document the medication administration, any drainage noted to come from vagina, and the condition of the skin in the perineal area. Medication documentation may be performed on the CMAR.	

Skill Checklists to Accompany Taylor's Clinical Nursing Skills:
A Nursing Process Approach

Name _____ Date _____

Unit _____ Position _____

Instructor/Evaluator: _____ Position _____

SKILL 5-19

Applying an Insulin Pump

Goal: To attach the insulin pump to successfully administer medication

Excellent	Satisfactory	Needs Practice		Comments
___	___	___	1. Bring equipment to patient's bedside. Check physician's order.	
___	___	___	2. Identify the person by checking the identification band on the patient's wrist and asking the patient his or her name.	
___	___	___	3. Explain the procedure to the patient. Provide privacy.	
___	___	___	4. Perform hand hygiene.	
___	___	___	5. Attach blunt ended needle or small-gauged needle to syringe. Follow Skill 5-3 to remove insulin from vial. Remove enough insulin to last patient 2 to 3 days plus 30 units for priming tubing.	
___	___	___	6. Attach sterile tubing to syringe. Push plunger of syringe until insulin is coming from introducer needle. Check for any bubbles in tubing.	
___	___	___	7. Program pump according to manufacturer's recommendations following physician's orders. Open the pump and place syringe in compartment according to manufacturer's directions. Close pump.	
___	___	___	8. Activate the insertion device. Place the needle between the prongs of the insertion device with sharp edge facing out. Push insertion set down until click is heard.	
___	___	___	9. Clean the area around the injection site with an antimicrobial swab. Use a firm circular motion while moving outward from the insertion site. Allow the antiseptic to dry.	
___	___	___	10. Remove the paper from the adhesive backing. Remove needle guard. Pinch skin at insertion site, press insertion device on the site, and press the release buttons to insert needle. Remove triggering device.	
___	___	___	11. While holding needle hub, turn it ¼ turn and remove needle. Discard appropriately.	
___	___	___	12. Apply sterile occlusive dressing over insertion site. Attach the pump to patient's clothing.	
___	___	___	13. Perform hand hygiene.	
___	___	___	14. Document type of insulin, pump settings, insertion site, and any teaching done with patient.	
___	___	___	15. Evaluate the patient's response to medication within the appropriate time frame.	

Skill Checklists to Accompany Taylor's Clinical Nursing Skills:
A Nursing Process Approach

Name _____ Date _____

Unit _____ Position _____

Instructor/Evaluator: _____ Position _____

SKILL 6-1
Preoperative Patient Care: Hospitalized Patient

Goal: To provide the necessary physical and psychological preparation for surgery.

Excellent	Satisfactory	Needs Practice		Comments
___	___	___	1. Identify patients for whom surgery is a greater risk:	
___	___	___	a. Very young or elderly patients	
___	___	___	b. Obese or malnourished patients	
___	___	___	c. Patients with fluid and electrolyte imbalances	
___	___	___	d. Patients in poor general health from chronic diseases and infectious processes	
___	___	___	e. Patients taking certain medications (ie, anticoagulants, antibiotics, diuretics, depressants, steroids)	
___	___	___	f. Patients who are extremely anxious	
___	___	___	2. Review nursing database, history, and physical examination. Check that baseline data are recorded; report those that are abnormal.	
___	___	___	3. Check that diagnostic testing has been completed and results are available; identify and report abnormal results.	
___	___	___	4. Promote optimal nutritional and hydration status.	
___	___	___	5. Identify learning needs of patient and family.	
___	___	___	6. Conduct preoperative teaching regarding coughing and deep-breathing exercises with splinting if necessary.	
___	___	___	7. Conduct preoperative teaching regarding respiratory therapy regimens, such as incentive spirometry.	
___	___	___	8. Conduct preoperative teaching regarding pain management after surgery.	
___	___	___	9. Conduct preoperative teaching regarding leg exercises.	
___	___	___	10. Provide preoperative teaching regarding early ambulation and turning in bed.	
___	___	___	11. Provide preoperative teaching regarding postoperative equipment and monitoring devices.	
___	___	___	12. Provide preoperative teaching regarding home care requirements.	
___	___	___	13. Document findings and instructions given.	
			Day Before Surgery	
___	___	___	14. Provide emotional support. Answer questions realistically. Provide with spiritual guidance if requested. Include family when possible.	

Excellent	Satisfactory	Needs Practice		
			## SKILL 6-1 ## Preoperative Patient Care: Hospitalized Patient ### (Continued)	
				Comments
___	___	___	15. Follow preoperative fluid and food restrictions.	
___	___	___	16. Prepare for elimination needs during and after surgery.	
___	___	___	17. Attend to patient's special hygiene needs (eg, use of antiseptic cleaning agents to prepare surgical site).	
___	___	___	18. Provide for adequate rest.	
			Day of Surgery	
___	___	___	19. Check that proper identification band is on patient.	
___	___	___	20. Check that preoperative consent forms are signed, witnessed, and correct; that advanced directives are in the medical record (as applicable); and that the medical record is in order.	
___	___	___	21. Check vital signs. Notify physician of any pertinent changes (eg, rise or drop in blood pressure, elevated temperature, cough, symptoms of infection).	
___	___	___	22. Provide hygiene and oral care. Remind patient of food and fluid restrictions and time when oral intake is restricted for surgery.	
___	___	___	23. Continue nutritional and hydration preparation.	
___	___	___	24. Remove cosmetics, jewelry, nail polish, and prostheses (eg, contact lenses, false eyelashes, dentures). Assess for loose teeth.	
___	___	___	25. Place valuables in appropriate area. Hospital safe is most appropriate place for valuables. They should not be placed in narcotics drawer.	
___	___	___	26. Have patient empty bladder and bowel before surgery.	
___	___	___	27. Attend to any special preoperative orders.	
___	___	___	28. Complete preoperative checklist and record patient's preoperative preparation.	
___	___	___	29. Administer preoperative medication as prescribed by physician/anesthesia provider.	
___	___	___	30. Raise the side rails of the bed; place the bed in the lowest position. Instruct the patient to remain in bed or on the stretcher. If necessary, a safety restraint may be used.	
___	___	___	31. Help move the patient from the bed to the transport stretcher if necessary. Reconfirm patient identification and ensure that all preoperative events and measures are documented.	
___	___	___	32. After the patient leaves for the operating room, prepare the room and bed for postoperative care. Anticipate any necessary equipment based on the type of surgery and the patient's history.	

Skill Checklists to Accompany Taylor's Clinical Nursing Skills:
A Nursing Process Approach

Name _____ Date _____

Unit _____ Position _____

Instructor/Evaluator: _____ Position _____

Excellent	Satisfactory	Needs Practice	SKILL 6-2 **Postoperative Care when Patient Returns to Room** **Goal:** To provide the necessary physical and psychological care after surgery.	Comments
⎯⎯	⎯⎯	⎯⎯	1. Upon return from PACU, obtain report from PACU nurse and review the operating room and PACU data. Check patient's identification. Perform hand hygiene. Place patient in safe position (semi- or high Fowler's or side lying). Note level of consciousness.	
⎯⎯	⎯⎯	⎯⎯	2. Monitor and record vital signs frequently. Assessment order may vary, but usual frequency includes taking vital signs every 15 minutes the first hour, every 30 minutes the next 2 hours, every hour for 4 hours, and, finally, every 4 hours.	
⎯⎯	⎯⎯	⎯⎯	3. Provide for warmth, using blankets as necessary. Assess skin color and condition.	
⎯⎯	⎯⎯	⎯⎯	4. Check dressings for color, odor, and amount of drainage. Feel under patient for bleeding.	
⎯⎯	⎯⎯	⎯⎯	5. Verify that all tubes and drains are patent and equipment is operative. Note amount of drainage in collection device.	
⎯⎯	⎯⎯	⎯⎯	6. Maintain intravenous infusion at correct rate.	
⎯⎯	⎯⎯	⎯⎯	7. Provide for a safe environment. Keep bed in low position with side rails up. Have call bell within patient's reach.	
⎯⎯	⎯⎯	⎯⎯	8. Relieve pain by administering medications ordered by physician. Check record to verify if analgesic medication was administered in PACU.	
⎯⎯	⎯⎯	⎯⎯	9. Record assessments and interventions on chart.	
			Ongoing Care	
⎯⎯	⎯⎯	⎯⎯	10. Promote optimal respiratory function.	
⎯⎯	⎯⎯	⎯⎯	a. Encourage coughing and deep breathing.	
⎯⎯	⎯⎯	⎯⎯	b. Perform incentive spirometry.	
⎯⎯	⎯⎯	⎯⎯	c. Encourage early ambulation.	
⎯⎯	⎯⎯	⎯⎯	d. Assist with frequent position change.	

Postoperative Care when
Patient Returns to Room *(Continued)*

Excellent	Satisfactory	Needs Practice		Comments
___	___	___	e. Administer oxygen as ordered.	
___	___	___	11. Maintain adequate circulation.	
___	___	___	a. Assist with frequent position changes.	
___	___	___	b. Encourage early ambulation.	
___	___	___	c. Apply antiembolic stockings or pneumatic compression devices if ordered by physician.	
___	___	___	d. Assist with leg and range-of-motion exercises if not contraindicated.	
___	___	___	12. Assess urinary elimination status.	
___	___	___	a. Promote voiding by offering bedpan at regular intervals.	
___	___	___	b. Monitor catheter drainage if present.	
___	___	___	c. Measure intake and output.	
___	___	___	13. Promote optimal nutrition status and return of gastrointestinal function.	
___	___	___	a. Assess for return of peristalsis.	
___	___	___	b. Assist with diet progression.	
___	___	___	c. Encourage fluid intake.	
___	___	___	d. Monitor intake.	
___	___	___	e. Medicate for nausea and vomiting as ordered by physician.	
___	___	___	14. Promote wound healing by using surgical asepsis. Assess condition of wound and any drainage.	
___	___	___	15. Provide for rest and comfort.	
___	___	___	16. Provide emotional support and spiritual support.	
___	___	___	17. Document findings and interventions used.	

Skill Checklists to Accompany Taylor's Clinical Nursing Skills:
A Nursing Process Approach

Name _____   Date _____

Unit _____   Position _____

Instructor/Evaluator: _____   Position _____

Excellent	Satisfactory	Needs Practice	SKILL 6-3 **Applying a Forced-Air Warming Device** **Goal:** To help the patient return to and maintain a temperature of 36.5° to 37.5°C (97.7° to 99.5°F).	Comments
____	____	____	1. Gather equipment. Check physician's order and explain procedure to patient.	
____	____	____	2. Perform hand hygiene.	
____	____	____	3. Assess temperature and document.	
____	____	____	4. Plug forced-air warming device into an electrical outlet. Place blanket over patient, with plastic side up. Keep air hose inlet at the foot of the patient's bed.	
____	____	____	5. Securely insert air hose to inlet. Place a lightweight fabric blanket over forced-air blanket. Turn machine on and adjust temperature of air to desired effect.	
____	____	____	6. Monitor the patient's temperature at least every 30 minutes while using the forced-air device. If rewarming a patient with hypothermia, do not raise temperature more than 1°C per hour to prevent a rapid vasodilation effect.	
____	____	____	7. Discontinue use of forced-air device once patient's temperature is adequate and patient is able to maintain the temperature without assistance.	
____	____	____	8. Remove device and clean according to agency policy and manufacturer's instructions. Document patient's status.	

Skill Checklists to Accompany Taylor's Clinical Nursing Skills:
A Nursing Process Approach

Name _____ Date _____

Unit _____ Position _____

Instructor/Evaluator: _____ Position _____

Excellent	Satisfactory	Needs Practice	SKILL 7-1 **Giving a Bed Bath**	Comments
			Goal: To provide or assist with personal hygiene; the patient will be clean and fresh.	
____	____	____	1. Discuss procedure with patient. Assess patient's ability to assist in the bathing process and personal hygiene preferences. Review patient's chart for any limitations in physical activity.	
____	____	____	2. Bring necessary equipment to bedside stand or overbed table. Remove sequential compression devices and antiembolism stockings from lower extremities according to agency protocol.	
____	____	____	3. Close curtains around bed and close door to the room if possible.	
____	____	____	4. Offer patient a bedpan or urinal.	
____	____	____	5. Perform hand hygiene.	
____	____	____	6. Raise patient's bed to the high position.	
____	____	____	7. Lower the side rails nearer to you and assist patient to the side of the bed where you will work. Have patient lie on his or her back.	
____	____	____	8. Loosen top covers and remove all except top sheet. Place bath blanket over patient and then remove top sheet while patient holds bath blanket in place. If linen is to be reused, fold it over a chair. Place soiled linen in laundry bag.	
____	____	____	9. Assist patient with oral hygiene, as necessary, and as described in Skill 7-5.	
____	____	____	10. Remove patient's gown and keep bath blanket in place. If patient has an intravenous line and is not wearing a gown with snap sleeves, remove gown from other arm first. Lower intravenous container and pass gown over tubing and container. Rehang container and check drip rate.	
____	____	____	11. Raise side rail. Fill basin with a sufficient amount of comfortably warm (43° to 46°C [110° to 115°F]) water. Change as necessary throughout the bath. Lower side rail closer to you when you return to the bedside to begin the bath.	

Excellent	Satisfactory	Needs Practice	SKILL 7-1 **Giving a Bed Bath** *(Continued)*	
				Comments
___	___	___	12. Fold washcloth like a mitt on your hand so there are no loose ends.	
___	___	___	13. Lay towel across patient's chest and on top of bath blanket.	
___	___	___	14. With no soap on the washcloth, wipe one eye from inner part of the eye near the nose to the outer part. Rinse or turn cloth before washing other eye.	
___	___	___	15. Bathe the patient's face, neck, and ears, avoiding soap on the face if the patient prefers.	
___	___	___	16. Expose patient's far arm and place towel lengthwise under it. Using firm strokes, wash arm and axilla, rinse, and dry.	
___	___	___	17. Place folded towel on bed next to patient's hand and put basin on towel. Soak patient's hand in basin. Wash, rinse, and dry hand.	
___	___	___	18. Repeat Actions 16 and 17 for the arm near to you. (An option for a shorter nurse or one prone to back strain might be to bathe one side of patient and move to the other side of bed to complete the bath.)	
___	___	___	19. Spread towel across patient's chest. Lower bath blanket to patient's umbilical area. Wash, rinse, and dry patient's chest. Keep patient's chest covered with towel between the wash and rinse. Pay special attention to skin folds under patient's breasts.	
___	___	___	20. Lower bath blanket to patient's perineal area. Place towel over patient's chest.	
___	___	___	21. Wash, rinse, and dry patient's abdomen. Carefully inspect and cleanse umbilical area and any abdominal folds or creases.	
___	___	___	22. Return bath blanket to original position and expose the patient's far leg. Place towel under far leg. Using firm strokes, wash, rinse, and dry patient's leg from ankle to knee and knee to groin.	
___	___	___	23. Fold towel near patient's foot area and place basin on towel. Place patient's foot in basin while supporting patient's ankle and heel in your hand and leg in your arm. Wash, rinse, and dry, paying particular attention to area between toes.	
___	___	___	24. Repeat Actions 22 and 23 for other leg and foot.	
___	___	___	25. Make sure patient is covered with bath blanket. Change water and washcloth at this point or earlier if necessary. Assist patient onto his or her side.	

SKILL 7-1
Giving a Bed Bath *(Continued)*

Excellent	Satisfactory	Needs Practice		Comments
___	___	___	26. Assist patient to a prone or side-lying position. Position bath blanket and towel to expose only back and buttocks.	
___	___	___	27. Wash, rinse, and dry patient's back and buttocks area. Pay particular attention to cleansing between gluteal folds and observe for any indication of redness or skin breakdown in the sacral area.	
___	___	___	28. If not contraindicated, give patient a back massage, as described in Skill 10-1. Back massage may also be given after perineal care.	
___	___	___	29. Refill basin with clean water. Discard washcloth and towel.	
___	___	___	30. Clean patient's perineal area or set up patient so he or she can complete perineal self-care.	
___	___	___	31. Help patient put on a clean gown and attend to personal hygiene needs.	
___	___	___	32. Protect pillow with a towel and groom patient's hair.	
___	___	___	33. Change bed linens, as described in Skills 7-3 and 7-4. Remove gloves and perform hand hygiene. Dispose of soiled linens according to agency policy.	
___	___	___	34. Record any significant observations and communication on patient's chart.	

Skill Checklists to Accompany Taylor's Clinical Nursing Skills:
A Nursing Process Approach

Name _____ Date _____

Unit _____ Position _____

Instructor/Evaluator: _____ Position _____

Excellent	Satisfactory	Needs Practice	SKILL 7-2 **Applying and Removing Antiembolism Stockings**	
			Goal: To promote venous return from lower extremities with minimal discomfort to patient.	**Comments**
___	___	___	1. Explain the rationale for use of elastic stockings to patient.	
___	___	___	2. Perform hand hygiene.	
___	___	___	3. Assist patient to the supine position. If patient has been sitting or walking, it is necessary to have him or her lie down with legs and feet well elevated for at least 15 minutes before applying stockings.	
___	___	___	4. Provide privacy. Expose legs one at a time and powder lightly unless patient has dry skin. If skin is dry, a lotion may be used. Powders and lotions are not recommended by some manufacturers.	
___	___	___	5. Place hand inside stocking and grasp heel area securely. Turn stocking inside out to the heel area.	
___	___	___	6. Ease foot of stocking over patient's foot and heel. Check that patient's heel is centered in heel pocket of stocking.	
___	___	___	7. Using your fingers and thumbs, carefully grasp edge of stocking and pull it up smoothly over ankle and calf until entire stocking is turned right side out. Pull forward slightly on toe section. Repeat for other leg. Caution patient not to roll stockings partially down.	
___	___	___	8. Perform hand hygiene.	
			Removing Stockings	
___	___	___	9. To remove stocking, grasp top of stocking with your thumbs and fingers and smoothly pull stocking off inside out to heel. Support patient's foot and ease stocking over it.	
___	___	___	10. Remove stockings once every shift for 20 to 30 minutes. Wash and air dry as necessary (according to manufacturer's directions).	
___	___	___	11. Record application of elastic stockings as well as assessment of patient's circulatory status and skin condition.	

Skill Checklists to Accompany Taylor's Clinical Nursing Skills:
A Nursing Process Approach

Name _____   Date _____

Unit _____   Position _____

Instructor/Evaluator: _____   Position _____

Excellent	Satisfactory	Needs Practice	SKILL 7-3 **Making an Unoccupied Bed** **Goal:** To promote a comfortable bed environment when bed is unoccupied without injury to nurse or patient.	Comments
___	___	___	1. Perform hand hygiene.	
___	___	___	2. Assemble equipment and arrange on a bedside chair in the order in which items will be used.	
___	___	___	3. Adjust patient's bed to the high position and drop bed side rails.	
___	___	___	4. Disconnect call bell or any tubes from bed linens.	
___	___	___	5. Loosen all linen as you move around bed from the head of the bed on the far side to the head of the bed on the near side.	
___	___	___	6. Fold reusable linens, such as sheets, blankets or spread, in place on bed in fourths and then hang them over a clean chair.	
___	___	___	7. Snugly roll all soiled linen inside the bottom sheet and place directly into laundry hamper. Do not place them on floor or furniture. Do not hold soiled linens against your uniform.	
___	___	___	8. If possible, shift mattress up to the head of the bed.	
___	___	___	9. Place bottom sheet with its center fold in the center of the bed and high enough to have a sufficient amount of the sheet to tuck under the head of the mattress.	
___	___	___	10. Place drawsheet with its center fold in the center of the bed and position so it will be located under patient's midsection. If using a protective pad, place it over the drawsheet in the proper area. Not all agencies use drawsheets routinely. The nurse may decide to use one.	
___	___	___	11. Tuck bottom sheet securely under the head of the mattress on one side of the bed, making a corner according to agency policy. Using a fitted bottom sheet eliminates the need to miter corners. Tuck remaining bottom sheet and drawsheet securely under mattress. (At this point, before moving to the other side of the bed, top linens may be placed on the bed, unfolded, and secured, allowing the entire side of the bed to be completed at one time.)	

Excellent	**Satisfactory**	**Needs Practice**	SKILL 7-3 **Making an Unoccupied Bed** *(Continued)*
			Comments
___	___	___	12. Move to the other side of the bed to secure bottom sheet under the head of the mattress and miter the corner. Pull remainder of sheet tightly and tuck under mattress. Do the same for the drawsheet.
___	___	___	13. Place top sheet on bed with its center fold in the center of the bed and with the top of the sheet placed so that the hem is even with the head of the mattress. Unfold top sheet in place. Follow same procedure with top blanket or spread, placing upper edge about 6 inches below top of the sheet.
___	___	___	14. Tuck top sheet and blanket under foot of bed on the near side. Miter corners.
___	___	___	15. Fold upper 6 inches of the top sheet down over the spread and make a cuff.
___	___	___	16. Move to other side of bed and follow the same procedure for securing top sheets under the foot of the bed and making a cuff.
___	___	___	17. Place pillows on the bed. Open each pillowcase in the same manner as opening other linens. Gather pillowcase over one hand toward the closed end. Grasp pillow with hand inside the pillowcase. Keeping a firm hold on top of pillow, pull cover onto pillow.
___	___	___	18. Place pillow at the head of the bed with the open end facing toward the window.
___	___	___	19. Fan-fold or pie-fold top linens.
___	___	___	20. Secure signal device on the bed according to agency policy.
___	___	___	21. Adjust bed to the low position.
___	___	___	22. Dispose of soiled linen according to agency policy. Perform hand hygiene.

Skill Checklists to Accompany Taylor's Clinical Nursing Skills:
A Nursing Process Approach

Name _____   Date _____

Unit _____   Position _____

Instructor/Evaluator: _____   Position _____

SKILL 7-4

Making an Occupied Bed

Goal: To provide a comfortable bed environment when bed is occupied without injury to the patient or nurse.

Excellent	Satisfactory	Needs Practice		Comments
____	____	____	1. Explain procedure to patient. Check patient's chart for limitations on patient's physical activity.	
____	____	____	2. Perform hand hygiene.	
____	____	____	3. Assemble equipment and arrange on bedside chair in the order items will be used.	
____	____	____	4. Close door or curtain.	
____	____	____	5. Adjust patient's bed to the high position. Lower side rail nearest you, leaving opposite side rail up. Place bed in the flat position unless contraindicated.	
____	____	____	6. Check bed linens for patient's personal items and disconnect call bell or any tubes from bed linens.	
____	____	____	7. Place a bath blanket, if available, over patient. Have patient hold onto bath blanket while you reach under it and remove top linens. Leave top sheet in place if a bath blanket is not used. Fold linen that is to be reused over the back of a chair. Discard soiled linen in laundry bag or hamper.	
____	____	____	8. If possible and if another person is available to assist, grasp mattress securely and shift it up to the head of the bed.	
____	____	____	9. Assist patient to turn toward the opposite side of the bed and reposition pillow under patient's head.	
____	____	____	10. Loosen all bottom linens from the head and sides of the bed.	
____	____	____	11. Fan-fold soiled linens as close to patient as possible.	
____	____	____	12. Using clean linen, make the near side of bed following Actions 9, 10, and 11 of Skill 7-3. Fan-fold clean linen as close to patient as possible.	
____	____	____	13. Raise side rail. Assist patient to roll over the folded linen in the middle of the bed toward you. Move to other side of bed and lower side rail.	
____	____	____	14. Loosen and remove all bottom linen. Place in a linen bag or hamper. Hold soiled linen away from your uniform.	

Excellent	Satisfactory	Needs Practice	SKILL 7-4 **Making an Occupied Bed** *(Continued)*	
				Comments
___	___	___	15. Ease the clean linen from under the patient. Pull taut and secure bottom sheet under the head of the mattress. Miter corners. Pull side of the sheet taut and tuck under side of the mattress. Repeat this with drawsheet.	
___	___	___	16. Assist patient to return to the center of the bed. Remove pillow and change pillowcases before replacing with open end facing the window.	
___	___	___	17. Apply top linen so that it is centered and top hems are even with the head of the mattress. Have patient hold onto the top linen so bath blanket can be removed.	
___	___	___	18. Secure top linens under foot of mattress and miter corners. Loosen top linens over patient's feet by grasping them in the area of the feet and pulling gently toward the foot of the bed.	
___	___	___	19. Raise side rail. Lower bed height and adjust head of the bed to a comfortable position. Reattach call bell and drainage tubes.	
___	___	___	20. Dispose of soiled linens according to agency policy. Perform hand hygiene.	

Skill Checklists to Accompany Taylor's Clinical Nursing Skills:
A Nursing Process Approach

Name _____ Date _____

Unit _____ Position _____

Instructor/Evaluator: _____ Position _____

Excellent	Satisfactory	Needs Practice	SKILL 7-5 **Assisting the Patient with Oral Care**	
			Goal: To assist with mechanical cleaning of oral cavity.	**Comments**
___	___	___	1. Explain procedure to patient.	
___	___	___	2. Perform hand hygiene. Don disposable gloves if assisting with oral care.	
___	___	___	3. Assemble equipment on overbed table within patient's reach.	
___	___	___	4. Provide privacy for patient.	
___	___	___	5. Lower side rail and assist patient to sitting position, if permitted, or turn patient onto the side. Place towel across patient's chest. Raise bed to a comfortable working position.	
___	___	___	6. Encourage patient to brush own teeth or assist if necessary.	
___	___	___	a. Moisten toothbrush and apply toothpaste to bristles.	
___	___	___	b. Place brush at a 45-degree angle to gum line and brush from gum line to crown of each tooth. Brush outer and inner surfaces. Brush back and forth across biting surface of each tooth.	
___	___	___	c. Brush tongue gently with toothbrush.	
___	___	___	d. Have patient rinse vigorously with water and spit into emesis basin. Repeat until clear. Suction may be used as an alternative for removing fluid and secretions from mouth.	
___	___	___	e. Assist patient to floss teeth, if necessary.	
___	___	___	f. Offer mouthwash if patient prefers.	
___	___	___	7. Assist the patient with removal and cleansing of dentures if necessary.	
___	___	___	a. Apply gentle pressure with 4 × 4 gauze to grasp and remove upper denture plate. Place it immediately in denture cup. Lift lower denture using slight rocking motion, remove, and place in denture cup.	
___	___	___	b. If patient prefers, add denture cleanser with water in a cup and follow preparation directions or brush all areas	

Assisting the Patient with Oral Care (*Continued*)

Excellent	Satisfactory	Needs Practice		Comments

thoroughly with toothbrush and paste. Place paper towels or washcloth in sink while brushing.

___ ___ ___   c. Rinse thoroughly with water and return dentures to patient.

___ ___ ___   d. Offer mouthwash so patient can rinse mouth before replacing dentures.

___ ___ ___   e. Apply lubricant to lips if necessary.

Flossing Teeth

___ ___ ___   8. Remove approximately 6 inches of dental floss from container or use a plastic floss holder. Wrap the floss around the index fingers keeping about 1 to $1\frac{1}{2}$ inches of floss taut between the fingers.

___ ___ ___   9. Insert the floss gently between the teeth, moving the floss back and forth and downward to the gums.

___ ___ ___   10. The floss should be moved up and down first on one side of a tooth and then on the side of the other tooth until the surfaces are clean.

___ ___ ___   11. Repeat actions 9 and 10 in the spaces between all teeth.

___ ___ ___   12. Instruct patient to rinse mouth well with water after flossing.

___ ___ ___   13. Remove equipment and assist patient to a position of comfort. Record any unusual bleeding or inflammation. Raise side rail and lower bed.

___ ___ ___   14. Remove disposable gloves from inside out and discard appropriately. Perform hand hygiene.

Skill Checklists to Accompany Taylor's Clinical Nursing Skills:
A Nursing Process Approach

Name _____   Date _____

Unit _____   Position _____

Instructor/Evaluator: _____   Position _____

Excellent	Satisfactory	Needs Practice	SKILL 7-6 **Providing Oral Care for the Dependent Patient**	
			Goal: To provide mechanical cleaning of oral cavity for a helpless patient; patient's mouth will be clean.	**Comments**
——	——	——	1. Explain procedure to patient.	
——	——	——	2. Perform hand hygiene and don disposable gloves.	
——	——	——	3. Assemble equipment on overbed table within reach.	
——	——	——	4. Provide privacy for patient. Adjust bed height to a comfortable position. Lower one side rail and position patient on the side with the head tilted forward. Place towel across patient's chest and emesis basin in position under chin.	
——	——	——	5. Open patient's mouth and gently insert a padded tongue blade between back molars if necessary.	
——	——	——	6. If teeth are present, brush carefully with toothbrush and paste. Remove dentures, if present, and clean before replacing (see Skill 7-5, Action 7). Use a toothette or gauze-padded tongue blade moistened with normal saline or diluted mouthwash solution to gently cleanse gums, mucous membranes, and tongue.	
——	——	——	7. Use gauze-padded tongue blade dipped in mouthwash solution to rinse oral cavity. If desired, insert rubber tip of irrigating syringe into patient's mouth and rinse gently with a small amount of water. Position patient's head to allow for return of water or use suction apparatus to remove the water from oral cavity.	
——	——	——	8. Apply lubricant to patient's lips.	
——	——	——	9. Remove equipment and return patient to a comfortable position. Raise side rail and lower bed. Record any unusual bleeding or inflammation.	
——	——	——	10. Perform hand hygiene.	

Skill Checklists to Accompany Taylor's Clinical Nursing Skills:
A Nursing Process Approach

Name _____   Date _____

Unit _____   Position _____

Instructor/Evaluator: _____   Position _____

Excellent	Satisfactory	Needs Practice	SKILL 7-7 **Giving a Bed Shampoo**	
			Goal: To clean patient's hair.	**Comments**
___	___	___	1. Gather equipment and place at bedside.	
___	___	___	2. Perform hand hygiene. If you suspect any cuts of the scalp or blood in the hair, don disposable gloves. Lower head of bed.	
___	___	___	3. Remove patient's pillow and place protective pad under patient's head and shoulders.	
___	___	___	4. Fill the pitcher with warm water (between 43° and 46°C [110° to 115°F]). Place shampoo board underneath patient's head by having patient lift the head.	
___	___	___	5. Place bucket on floor underneath the drain of the shampoo board.	
___	___	___	6. Pour pitcher of warm water slowly over patient's head, making sure that all hair is saturated. Refill pitcher if needed.	
___	___	___	7. Apply a small amount of shampoo to the patient's hair. Massage deep into the scalp, being careful to avoid any cuts, lesions, or sore spots.	
___	___	___	8. Rinse with warm water (between 43° and 46°C [110° to 115°F]) until all shampoo is out of hair. Repeat shampoo if necessary.	
___	___	___	9. If patient has thick hair or requests, apply a small amount of conditioner to the hair and massage throughout. Avoid any cuts, lesions, or sore spots.	
___	___	___	10. If bucket is small, empty before rinsing hair. Rinse with warm water (between 43° and 46°C [110° to 115°F]) until all conditioner is out of hair.	
___	___	___	11. Place towel around patient's hair. Remove shampoo board.	
___	___	___	12. Pat dry hair being careful to avoid any cuts, lesions, or sore spots. Remove protective padding but keep one dry protective pad under patient's hair.	
___	___	___	13. Gently brush hair, removing any tangles as needed.	
___	___	___	14. Blow dry hair on a cool setting if allowed and if patient wishes.	
___	___	___	15. Change patient's gown and remove protective pad.	
___	___	___	16. Remove gloves. Perform hand hygiene.	
___	___	___	17. Document hair wash and any cuts or lesions that are found.	

Name _____ Date _____

Unit _____ Position _____

Instructor/Evaluator: _____ Position _____

SKILL 7-8
Removing and Cleaning Contact Lenses

Excellent	Satisfactory	Needs Practice	**Goal:** To clean lenses without causing trauma to the eye.	Comments
——	——	——	1. Explain procedure to patient.	
——	——	——	2. Perform hand hygiene. Don disposable gloves.	
——	——	——	3. Assist the patient to the supine position. Elevate the bed. Lower the side rail closest to you.	
——	——	——	4. If containers are not already labeled, do so now. Place 5 mL of normal saline in each container.	
			Removing Hard Contact Lenses	
——	——	——	5. If the lens is not centered over the cornea, apply gentle pressure on the lower eyelid to center the lens.	
——	——	——	6. Gently pull the outer corner of the eye toward the ear.	
——	——	——	7. Position the other hand below the lens and ask the patient to blink.	
——	——	——	8. Gently spread the eyelids beyond the top and bottom edges of the lens.	
——	——	——	9. Gently press the lower eyelid up against the bottom of the lens.	
——	——	——	10. After the lens is tipped slightly, move the eyelids toward one another to cause the lens to slide out between the eyelids.	
			If a Suction Cup Remover Is Available	
——	——	——	11. Ensure that contact lens is centered on cornea. Place a drop of sterile saline on the suction cup.	
——	——	——	12. Place the suction cup in the center of the contact lens and gently pull the contact lens off of the eye.	
——	——	——	13. To remove the suction cup from the lens, slide the lens off sideways.	
——	——	——	14. Have the patient look forward. Retract the lower lid with one hand. Using the pad of the index finger of the other hand, move the lens down to the sclera.	
——	——	——	15. Using the pads of the thumb and index finger, grasp the lens with a gentle pinching motion and remove.	

Excellent	Satisfactory	Needs Practice	SKILL 7-8 **Removing and Cleaning Contact Lenses** *(Continued)*	Comments
			If Rubber Pincer Is Available	
___	___	___	16. Visualize the placement of the contact and place the rubber pincers in the center of the lens.	
___	___	___	17. Gently squeeze the pincers and remove the lens from the eye.	
___	___	___	18. Place removed contact into the appropriately marked container. Repeat actions to remove other contact.	
___	___	___	19. If patient is awake and has glasses at bedside, offer patient glasses.	
___	___	___	20. Remove gloves. Perform hand hygiene.	
___	___	___	21. Document the removal of contact lenses as well as the condition of the eye: drainage, color of sclera, and/or complaints of pain.	

Skill Checklists to Accompany Taylor's Clinical Nursing Skills:
A Nursing Process Approach

Name _____ Date _____

Unit _____ Position _____

Instructor/Evaluator: _____ Position _____

Excellent	Satisfactory	Needs Practice	SKILL 7-9 **Assisting with a Sitz Bath**	Comments
			Goal: The patient will state an increase in comfort.	
⸺	⸺	⸺	1. Explain the procedure to the patient.	
⸺	⸺	⸺	2. Perform hand hygiene and don disposable gloves.	
⸺	⸺	⸺	3. Assemble equipment in bathroom.	
⸺	⸺	⸺	4. Raise lid of toilet. Place bowl of sitz bath with drainage ports to rear and infusion port in front in the toilet. Fill bowl of sitz bath about half of the way full with tepid to warm water (37° to 46°C [98° to 115°F]).	
⸺	⸺	⸺	5. Clamp tubing on bag. Fill bag with same temperature water as mentioned above. Hang bag above shoulder height of the patient on hook or intravenous pole.	
⸺	⸺	⸺	6. Assist patient to sit on toilet. Insert tubing into infusion port of sitz bath. Slowly unclamp tubing and allow sitz bath to fill.	
⸺	⸺	⸺	7. Clamp tubing once sitz bath is full. Instruct patient to open clamp when water in bowl becomes cool. Ensure that call bell is within reach. Instruct patient to call if he or she feels light headed, spacey, dizzy, or has any other problems. Patient should be instructed not to try standing without assistance.	
⸺	⸺	⸺	8. When patient is through with sitz bath, help patient to stand and gently pat bottom dry. Assist patient to bed or chair. Ensure that call bell is within reach.	
⸺	⸺	⸺	9. Empty and disinfect sitz bath bowl according to agency policy. Remove gloves and perform hand hygiene.	
⸺	⸺	⸺	10. Document the sitz bath, including water temperature, length of sitz bath, and how patient tolerated sitz bath.	

Name _____   Date _____

Unit _____   Position _____

Instructor/Evaluator: _____   Position _____

Excellent	Satisfactory	Needs Practice	SKILL 7-10 **Assisting the Patient to Shave**	Comments
			Goal: To ensure the patient will be clean without evidence of any hair growth or trauma to the skin.	
___	___	___	1. Gather equipment. Explain procedure to patient.	
___	___	___	2. Perform hand hygiene and don disposable gloves.	
___	___	___	3. Fill bath basin with warm (between 43° and 46°C [110° to 115°F]) water. Take wash cloth and moisten the area to be shaved.	
___	___	___	4. Dispense shaving cream into palm of hand. Rub hands together and then apply in a layer around ½-inch thick to area to be shaved.	
___	___	___	5. Using a smooth stroke, begin shaving. Pull the skin so that it is taut if necessary. If shaving the face, shave with the hair in downward short strokes. If shaving a leg, shave against the hair in upward short strokes.	
___	___	___	6. Wash the patient's skin of residual shaving cream.	
___	___	___	7. If patient requests, apply aftershave or lotion to area shaved.	
___	___	___	8. Remove gloves, discard, and perform hand hygiene.	

Skill Checklists to Accompany Taylor's Clinical Nursing Skills:
A Nursing Process Approach

Name _____ Date _____

Unit _____ Position _____

Instructor/Evaluator: _____ Position _____

SKILL 8-1
Removing Sutures

Goal: To remove sutures without contaminating the incisional area, causing trauma to the wound, or causing patient pain or discomfort.

Excellent	Satisfactory	Needs Practice		Comments
___	___	___	1. Review the physician's order for suture removal.	
___	___	___	2. Gather the necessary supplies.	
___	___	___	3. Identify the patient. Explain the procedure to the patient. Describe the sensation that will be experienced as a pulling or slightly uncomfortable experience.	
___	___	___	4. Perform hand hygiene.	
___	___	___	5. Close the room door or curtains. Place the bed at an appropriate and comfortable working height.	
___	___	___	6. Assist the patient to a comfortable position that provides easy access to the wound area. Use a bath blanket to cover any exposed area other than the wound.	
___	___	___	7. Put on gloves. Remove and dispose of any dressings on the surgical incision. Remove gloves and put on a new pair. Inspect the incision area.	
___	___	___	8. Clean the incision using the wound cleanser and gauze, according to facility policy and procedure.	
___	___	___	9. Using the sterile forceps, grasp the knot of the first suture and gently lift the knot up off the skin.	
___	___	___	10. Using the sterile scissors, cut one side of the suture below the knot close to the skin. Grasp the knot with the forceps and pull the cut suture through the skin. Be sure to avoid pulling the visible portion of the suture through the underlying tissue.	
___	___	___	11. Proceed to remove every other suture to be sure the wound edges are healed. If they are, remove the remaining sutures as ordered.	
___	___	___	12. Apply Steri-Strips, if ordered. If necessary, prepare skin with tincture of benzoin before applying Steri-Strips.	
___	___	___	13. Reapply the dressing, depending on the physician's orders and facility policy.	
___	___	___	14. Remove gloves and perform hand hygiene.	
___	___	___	15. Document the procedure and assessments.	

Skill Checklists to Accompany Taylor's Clinical Nursing Skills:
A Nursing Process Approach

Name _____   Date _____

Unit _____   Position _____

Instructor/Evaluator: _____   Position _____

Excellent	Satisfactory	Needs Practice	SKILL 8-2 **Removing Surgical Staples**	Comments
			Goal: To remove staples without contaminating the incisional area, without causing trauma to the wound, and without causing patient pain or discomfort.	
____	____	____	1. Review the physician's order for staple removal.	
____	____	____	2. Gather the necessary supplies.	
____	____	____	3. Identify the patient. Explain the procedure to the patient. Describe the sensation that will be experienced as a pulling or slightly uncomfortable experience.	
____	____	____	4. Perform hand hygiene.	
____	____	____	5. Close the room door or curtains. Place the bed at an appropriate and comfortable working height.	
____	____	____	6. Assist the patient to a comfortable position that provides easy access to the wound area. Use a bath blanket to cover any exposed area other than the wound.	
____	____	____	7. Put on gloves. Remove and dispose of any dressings on the surgical incision using proper technique. Remove gloves and put on a new pair.	
____	____	____	8. Clean the incision using the wound cleanser and gauze, according to facility policy and procedure.	
____	____	____	9. Position the sterile staple remover under the staple to be removed. Firmly close the staple remover. The staple will bend in the middle and the edges will pull up out of the skin.	
____	____	____	10. Proceed to remove every other staple to be sure the wound edges are healed. If they are, remove the remaining staples as ordered.	
____	____	____	11. Apply Steri-Strips, according to facility policy or physician's order. Prepare skin with tincture of benzoin if indicated.	
____	____	____	12. Reapply the dressing, depending on the physician's orders and facility policy.	
____	____	____	13. Remove gloves and perform hand hygiene.	
____	____	____	14. Document the procedure and assessments.	

Skill Checklists to Accompany Taylor's Clinical Nursing Skills:
A Nursing Process Approach

Name _____ Date _____

Unit _____ Position _____

Instructor/Evaluator: _____ Position _____

Excellent	Satisfactory	Needs Practice	SKILL 8-3 **Caring for a Penrose Drain**	Comments
			Goal: To keep Penrose drain patent and intact; care is performed without contaminating the wound area, causing trauma to the wound, or causing patient pain or discomfort.	
___	___	___	1. Review the physician's order for drain and site care or the nursing plan of care related to drain care.	
___	___	___	2. Gather the necessary supplies.	
___	___	___	3. Identify the patient. Explain the procedure to the patient. Inquire about any known allergies, specifically related to the products being used for wound care.	
___	___	___	4. Perform hand hygiene.	
___	___	___	5. Close the room door or curtains. Place the bed at an appropriate and comfortable working height.	
___	___	___	6. Place a waste receptacle at a convenient location for use during the procedure.	
___	___	___	7. Assist the patient to a comfortable position that provides easy access to the drain area. Use a bath blanket to cover any exposed area other than the drain. If necessary, place a waterproof pad under the drain site.	
___	___	___	8. Check the position of the drain or drains before removing the dressing. Put on the clean disposable gloves and loosen tape on the old dressings. Use an adhesive remover to help get the tape off, if necessary.	
___	___	___	9. Carefully remove the soiled dressings. If any part of the dressing sticks to the underlying skin, use small amounts of sterile saline to help loosen and remove. Do not reach over the drain site.	
___	___	___	10. After removing the dressing, note the presence, amount, type, color, and odor of any drainage on the dressings. Place soiled dressings in the appropriate waste receptacle. Remove gloves and dispose of in appropriate waste receptacle.	
___	___	___	11. Inspect the drain site for appearance and drainage. Assess if any pain is present. Closely observe the safety pin in the drain. Note any problems to include in your documentation.	
___	___	___	12. If the pin or drain is crusted, replace the pin with a new sterile pin. Take care not to dislodge the drain.	

Excellent	Satisfactory	Needs Practice	SKILL 8-3 **Caring for a Penrose Drain** *(Continued)*	
				Comments
——	——	——	13. Using sterile technique, prepare a sterile work area and open the needed supplies.	
——	——	——	14. Open the sterile cleaning solution. Pour the cleansing solution into the basin. Add the gauze sponges.	
——	——	——	15. Put on sterile gloves.	
——	——	——	16. Cleanse the drain site with the cleansing solution. Use forceps and moistened gauze or cotton-tipped applicators. Start at the drain insertion site, moving in a circular motion toward the periphery. Use each gauze sponge or applicator only once. Discard and use new gauze if additional cleansing is needed.	
——	——	——	17. Dry the skin with a new gauze pad. Place the drain sponge under the drain. Place several gauze pads around the drain site. Apply gauze pads over the drain.	
——	——	——	18. Apply ABD pads over the gauze. Remove gloves and dispose of them.	
——	——	——	19. Tape the ABD pads securely to the patient's skin.	
——	——	——	20. After securing the dressing, remove all remaining equipment, place the patient in a position of comfort with side rails up and bed in the lowest position, and perform hand hygiene.	
——	——	——	21. Record the procedure, wound assessment, and the patient's reaction to the procedure according to institution's guidelines.	
——	——	——	22. Check all dressings every shift. More frequent checking may be needed if a wound is more complex or dressings become saturated more frequently.	

Skill Checklists to Accompany Taylor's Clinical Nursing Skills:
A Nursing Process Approach

Name _____   Date _____

Unit _____   Position _____

Instructor/Evaluator: _____   Position _____

Excellent	Satisfactory	Needs Practice	SKILL 8-4 **Caring for a T-Tube Drain**	Comments
			Goal: To keep the T-Tube drain patent and intact; care is performed without contaminating the wound area, causing trauma to the wound, or causing patient pain or discomfort.	
____	____	____	1. Review the physician's order for drain and site care or the nursing plan of care related to drain care.	
____	____	____	2. Gather the necessary supplies.	
____	____	____	3. Identify the patient. Explain the procedure to the patient. Inquire about any known allergies, specifically related to the products being used for wound care.	
____	____	____	4. Perform hand hygiene.	
____	____	____	5. Close the room door or curtains. Place the bed at an appropriate and comfortable working height.	
____	____	____	6. Place a waste receptacle at a convenient location for use during the procedure.	
____	____	____	7. Assist the patient to a comfortable position that provides easy access to the drain area. Use a bath blanket to cover any exposed area other than the drain. Place a waterproof pad under the drain site.	
			Emptying Drainage	
____	____	____	8. Put on clean gloves.	
____	____	____	9. Using sterile technique, open a gauze pad, making a sterile field with the outer wrapper.	
____	____	____	10. Place the graduated collection container under the outlet valve of the drainage bag. Without contaminating the outlet valve, pull the cap off and empty the bag's contents completely into the container; use the gauze to wipe the valve, and reseal the outlet valve.	
____	____	____	11. Carefully measure and record the character, color, and amount of the drainage. Discard the drainage according to facility policy.	
____	____	____	12. Perform hand hygiene.	
			Cleaning the Drain Site	
____	____	____	13. Check the position of the drain or drains before removing the dressing. Put on clean disposable gloves and loosen tape on the old dressings. If necessary, use an adhesive remover to help get the tape off.	

Excellent	Satisfactory	Needs Practice	SKILL 8-4 **Caring for a T-Tube Drain** *(Continued)*	
				Comments
——	——	——	14. Carefully remove the soiled dressings. If any part of the dressing sticks to the underlying skin, use small amounts of sterile saline to help loosen and remove. Do not reach over the drain site.	
——	——	——	15. After removing the dressing, note the presence, amount, type, color, and odor of any drainage on the dressings. Place soiled dressings in the appropriate waste receptacle. Remove gloves and dispose of in appropriate waste receptacle.	
——	——	——	16. Inspect the drain site for appearance and drainage. Assess if any pain is present. Note any problems to include in your documentation.	
——	——	——	17. Using sterile technique, prepare a sterile work area and open the needed supplies.	
——	——	——	18. Open the sterile cleaning solution. Pour the cleansing solution into the basin. Add the gauze sponges.	
——	——	——	19. Put on sterile gloves.	
——	——	——	20. Cleanse the drain site with the cleansing solution. Use the forceps and the moistened gauze or cotton-tipped applicators. Start at the drain insertion site, moving in a circular motion toward the periphery. Use each gauze sponge only once. Discard and use new gauze if additional cleansing is needed.	
——	——	——	21. Allow the area to dry or dry with a new sterile gauze.	
——	——	——	22. Place the drain sponge under the drain. Place several gauze pads around the drain site. Apply gauze pads over the drain. Alternately, place the transparent dressing over the tube and dressings.	
——	——	——	23. Secure the dressings with tape as needed. Be careful not to kink the tubing.	
——	——	——	24. After securing the dressing, remove all remaining equipment, place the patient in a position of comfort with side rails up and bed in the lowest position, and perform hand hygiene.	
——	——	——	25. Record the procedure, your wound assessment, and the patient's reaction to the procedure using your institution's guidelines.	
——	——	——	26. Check all dressings every shift. More frequent checking may be needed if a wound is more complex or dressings become saturated quickly.	

Skill Checklists to Accompany Taylor's Clinical Nursing Skills:
A Nursing Process Approach

Name _____ Date _____

Unit _____ Position _____

Instructor/Evaluator: _____ Position _____

Excellent	Satisfactory	Needs Practice	SKILL 8-5 **Caring for a Jackson-Pratt Drain** **Goal:** To keep the drain remains and intact; care is performed without contaminating the wound area, causing trauma to the wound, or causing patient pain or discomfort.	Comments
___	___	___	1. Review the physician's order for drain and site care or the nursing plan of care related to drain care.	
___	___	___	2. Gather the necessary supplies.	
___	___	___	3. Identify the patient. Explain the procedure to the patient. Inquire about any known allergies, specifically related to the products being used for wound care.	
___	___	___	4. Perform hand hygiene.	
___	___	___	5. Close the room door or curtains. Place the bed at an appropriate and comfortable working height.	
___	___	___	6. Assist the patient to a comfortable position that provides easy access to the drain area. Use a bath blanket to cover any exposed area other than the drain. Place a waterproof pad under the drain site.	
___	___	___	7. Put on clean gloves; don mask or face shield if indicated.	
___	___	___	8. Place the graduated collection container under the outlet valve of the drain. Without contaminating the outlet valve, pull the cap off. The chamber will expand completely as it draws in air. Empty the chamber's contents completely into the container. Use the alcohol pad to clean the chamber's spout and cap. Fully compress the chamber with one hand and replace the plug with your other hand.	
___	___	___	9. Check the patency of the equipment. Make sure the tubing is free from twists and kinks.	
___	___	___	10. Secure the Jackson-Pratt drain to the patient's gown below the wound, making sure that there is no tension on the tubing.	
___	___	___	11. Carefully measure and record the character, color, and amount of the drainage. Discard the drainage according to facility policy.	
___	___	___	12. If the drain site has a dressing, redress the site as outlined in Skill 8-3.	

Excellent	Satisfactory	Needs Practice	SKILL 8-5 **Caring for a Jackson-Pratt Drain** *(Continued)*	Comments
___	___	___	13. If the drain site is open to air, observe the sutures that secure the drain to the patient's skin. Look for signs of pulling, tearing, swelling, or infection of the surrounding skin.	
___	___	___	14. Gently clean the sutures with the gauze pad soaked in normal saline. Dry with a new gauze pad.	
___	___	___	15. Remove gloves and all remaining equipment, place the patient in a position of comfort with side rails up and bed in the lowest position, and perform hand hygiene.	
___	___	___	16. Record the procedure, your wound assessment, and the patient's reaction to the procedure using your institution's guidelines.	

Skill Checklists to Accompany Taylor's Clinical Nursing Skills:
A Nursing Process Approach

Name _____ Date _____

Unit _____ Position _____

Instructor/Evaluator: _____ Position _____

Excellent	Satisfactory	Needs Practice	SKILL 8-6 **Caring for a Hemovac Drain** **Goal:** To keep the drain patent and intact; care is performed without contaminating the wound area, causing trauma to the wound, or causing patient pain or discomfort.	Comments
____	____	____	1. Review the physician's order for drain and site care or the nursing plan of care related to drain care.	
____	____	____	2. Gather the necessary supplies.	
____	____	____	3. Identify the patient. Explain the procedure to the patient. Inquire about any known allergies, specifically related to the products being used for wound care.	
____	____	____	4. Perform hand hygiene.	
____	____	____	5. Close the room door or curtains. Place the bed at an appropriate and comfortable working height.	
____	____	____	6. Assist the patient to a comfortable position that provides easy access to the drain area. Use a bath blanket to cover any exposed area other than the drain. Place a waterproof pad under the drain site.	
____	____	____	7. Put on clean gloves and other personal protective equipment, such as mask or face shield as necessary.	
____	____	____	8. Place the graduated collection container under the pouring spout of the drain. Without contaminating the outlet valve, uncap the valve. The chamber will expand completely as it draws in air. Empty the chamber's contents completely into the container. Use the alcohol pad to clean the chamber's spout and cap. Fully compress the chamber by pushing the top and bottom together with your hands. Keep the device tightly compressed while you reinsert the plug.	
____	____	____	9. Check the patency of the equipment. Make sure the tubing is free from twists and kinks.	
____	____	____	10. Secure the Hemovac drain to the patient's gown below the wound, making sure that there is no tension on the tubing.	
____	____	____	11. Carefully measure and record the character, color, and amount of the drainage. Discard the drainage according to facility policy.	
____	____	____	12. If the drain site has a dressing, redress the site as outlined in Skill 8-3.	

Excellent	Satisfactory	Needs Practice	SKILL 8-6 **Caring for a Hemovac Drain** *(Continued)*	Comments
____	____	____	13. If the drain site is open to air, observe the sutures that secure the drain to the patient's skin. Look for signs of pulling, tearing, swelling, or infection of the surrounding skin.	
____	____	____	14. Gently clean the sutures with the gauze pad soaked in normal saline. Dry with a new gauze pad.	
____	____	____	15. Remove gloves and all remaining equipment, place the patient in a position of comfort with side rails up and bed in the lowest position, and perform hand hygiene.	
____	____	____	16. Record the procedure, your wound assessment, and the patient's reaction to the procedure using your institution's guidelines	

Skill Checklists to Accompany Taylor's Clinical Nursing Skills:
A Nursing Process Approach

Name _____   Date _____

Unit _____   Position _____

Instructor/Evaluator: _____   Position _____

SKILL 8-7

Cleaning a Wound and Applying a Sterile Dressing

Goal: To promote wound healing and protect wound from injury.

Excellent	Satisfactory	Needs Practice		Comments
___	___	___	1. Review the physician's order for wound care of the nursing plan of care related to wound care.	
___	___	___	2. Gather the necessary supplies.	
___	___	___	3. Identify the patient. Explain the procedure to the patient. Inquire about any known allergies, specifically related to the products being used for wound care.	
___	___	___	4. Perform hand hygiene.	
___	___	___	5. Close door or curtain. Place the bed at an appropriate and comfortable working height.	
___	___	___	6. Place a waste receptacle or bag at a convenient location for use during the procedure.	
___	___	___	7. Assist patient to comfortable position that provides easy access to wound area. Use a bath blanket to cover any exposed area other than the wound. If necessary, place a waterproof pad under the wound site.	
___	___	___	8. Check the position of drains, tubes, or other adjuncts before removing the dressing. Put on the clean disposable gloves and loosen tape on the old dressings. If necessary, use an adhesive remover to help get the tape off.	
___	___	___	9. Carefully remove the soiled dressings. If any part of the dressing sticks to the underlying skin, use small amounts of sterile saline to help loosen and remove. Do not reach over the wound.	
___	___	___	10. After removing the dressing, note the presence, amount, type, color, and odor of any drainage on the dressings. Place soiled dressings in the appropriate waste receptacle. Remove your gloves and dispose of in appropriate waste receptacle.	
___	___	___	11. Inspect the wound site for appearance and drainage. Assess if any pain is present. Check the sutures, Steri-Strips, staples, and drains or tubes. Note any problems to include in your documentation.	
___	___	___	12. Using sterile technique, prepare a sterile work area and open the needed supplies.	

Excellent	Satisfactory	Needs Practice	SKILL 8-7 **Cleaning a Wound and Applying a Sterile Dressing** *(Continued)*	Comments
——	——	——	13. Open the sterile cleaning solution. Depending on the amount of cleaning needed, the solution might be poured directly over gauze sponges for small cleaning jobs or in a basin for more complex or larger cleaning.	
——	——	——	14. Put on sterile gloves.	
——	——	——	15. Clean the wound. If needed, use sterile forceps to clean the area. Clean the wound from top to bottom and from the center to the outside. Following this pattern, use gauze for each wipe, placing the used gauze in the waste receptacle. Do not touch any surface with the gloves or forceps.	
——	——	——	16. If a drain is in use, clean around the drain using a circular motion. Wipe from the center toward the outside. Use the gauze a single time and then dispose of it.	
——	——	——	17. Once the wound is cleansed, dry the area using a gauze sponge in the same manner. Apply ointment or any other treatments if ordered.	
——	——	——	18. Apply a layer of dry sterile dressing over the wound. Forceps may be used to apply the dressing.	
——	——	——	19. Place a second layer of gauze over the wound site.	
——	——	——	20. Apply a Surgi-Pad or ABD dressing over the gauze at the site as the outermost layer of the dressing.	
——	——	——	21. Remove and discard sterile gloves. It is often easier to apply the items used to secure the dressing in place when working without gloves. Apply tape or tie tapes to secure the dressings.	
——	——	——	22. After securing the dressing label dressing with date and time, remove all remaining equipment, place the patient in a position of comfort with side rails up and bed in the lowest position, and perform hand hygiene.	
——	——	——	23. Record the procedure, wound assessment, and the patient's reaction to the procedure according to institution's guidelines.	
——	——	——	24. Check all wound dressings every shift. More frequent checks may be needed if the wound is more complex or dressings become saturated quickly.	

Skill Checklists to Accompany Taylor's Clinical Nursing Skills:
A Nursing Process Approach

Name _____ Date _____

Unit _____ Position _____

Instructor/Evaluator: _____ Position _____

Excellent	Satisfactory	Needs Practice	SKILL 8-8 **Collecting a Wound Culture** **Goal:** To collect wound drainage for laboratory analysis of microorganisms that cause infection without exposing patient to additional pathogens.	Comments
___	___	___	1. Review the physician's order for obtaining a wound culture.	
___	___	___	2. Gather the necessary supplies.	
___	___	___	3. Identify the patient and check the specimen label to make sure the information matches. Explain the procedure to your patient.	
___	___	___	4. Perform hand hygiene.	
___	___	___	5. Close the room door or curtains. Place the bed at an appropriate and comfortable working height.	
___	___	___	6. Place an appropriate waste receptacle within easy reach for use during the procedure.	
___	___	___	7. Assist the patient to a comfortable position that provides easy access to the wound. If necessary, drape the patient with a bath blanket to expose only the wound area. Check the culture label again against the patient's identification bracelet.	
___	___	___	8. Put on the clean disposable gloves to remove any dressings. Loosen the tape and old dressings. Do not reach over the wound. Remove the dressing and dispose of it in the receptacle. Assess the wound and the characteristics of any drainage. Remove gloves and dispose of them.	
___	___	___	9. Set up sterile field with supplies if necessary. Put on the sterile gloves and clean the wound according to facility policy and procedure. Remove gloves and dispose of them.	
___	___	___	10. Twist the cap to loosen the swab on the Culturette tube or open the separate swab and remove the cap from the culture tube. Keep the swab and inside of culture tube sterile.	
___	___	___	11. Put on a clean glove or new sterile glove, if necessary.	
___	___	___	12. Carefully insert the swab into the wound and gently roll the swab to obtain a sample. Use another swab if collecting a specimen from another site.	

Excellent	Satisfactory	Needs Practice		Comments

SKILL 8-8

Collecting a Wound Culture *(Continued)*

Excellent	Satisfactory	Needs Practice		Comments
——	——	——	13. Place the swab back in the culture tube. Do not touch the outside of the tube with the swab. Then secure the cap. Some Culturette tubes have an ampule of medium at the bottom of the tube. It might be necessary to crush this ampule to activate. Follow the manufacturer's instructions for use.	
——	——	——	14. Remove your gloves and discard accordingly. Perform hand hygiene.	
——	——	——	15. Don sterile goves and replace the patient's dressing as needed following the appropriate procedure.	
——	——	——	16. Remove gloves and perform hand hygiene. Remove any equipment and leave the patient comfortable, with the side rails up and the bed in the lowest position.	
——	——	——	17. Complete labeling the specimen according to your institution's guidelines and send it to the laboratory in a biohazard bag.	
——	——	——	18. Document the procedure, the wound assessment, and the patient's reaction to the procedure following your institution's guidelines.	

Skill Checklists to Accompany Taylor's Clinical Nursing Skills:
A Nursing Process Approach

Name _____   Date _____

Unit _____   Position _____

Instructor/Evaluator: _____   Position _____

SKILL 8-9
Irrigating a Sterile Wound

Goal: To direct flow of solution into wound to clean area of pathogens and debris without causing contamination, trauma, or patient pain or discomfort.

Excellent	Satisfactory	Needs Practice		Comments
___	___	___	1. Review the physician's order for wound care or the nursing plan of care related to wound care.	
___	___	___	2. Gather the necessary supplies.	
___	___	___	3. Identify the patient and explain the procedure. Determine if there are allergies to any of the materials or solutions needed for the procedure.	
___	___	___	4. Perform hand hygiene.	
___	___	___	5. Close the room door or curtains. Place the bed at a comfortable working height.	
___	___	___	6. Assist the patient to a comfortable position that provides easy access to the wound area. Position the patient so the irrigation solution will flow from the upper end of the wound toward the lower end. Expose the area and drape the patient with a bath blanket if needed. Put a waterproof pad under the wound area to protect the bed.	
___	___	___	7. Have the disposal bag or waste receptacle within easy reach for use during the irrigation.	
___	___	___	8. Put on a gown, mask, and eye protection.	
___	___	___	9. Put on clean disposable gloves and remove the soiled dressings.	
___	___	___	10. Assess the wound for size, appearance, and drainage. Assess the appearance of the surrounding tissue.	
___	___	___	11. Discard the dressings in the receptacle. Remove your gloves and put them in the receptacle.	
___	___	___	12. Using sterile technique, prepare a sterile field and add all the sterile supplies needed for the procedure to the field. Pour warmed sterile irrigating solution into the sterile container.	
___	___	___	13. Put on sterile gloves.	
___	___	___	14. Position the sterile basin below the wound to collect the irrigation fluid.	
___	___	___	15. Fill the irrigation syringe with solution. Using your nondominant hand, gently apply pressure to the basin	

Excellent	Satisfactory	Needs Practice	SKILL 8-9 **Irrigating a Sterile Wound** *(Continued)*
			Comments

			against the skin below the wound to form a seal with the skin.	
___	___	___	16. Gently direct a stream of solution into the wound. Keep the tip of the syringe at least 1 inch above the upper tip of the wound. When using a catheter tip, insert it gently into the wound until it meets resistance. Gently flush all wound areas.	
___	___	___	17. Watch for the solution to flow smoothly and evenly. When the solution from the wound flows out clear, discontinue irrigation.	
___	___	___	18. Dry the surrounding skin with a sterile gauze sponge.	
___	___	___	19. Apply a new sterile dressing to the wound as previously discussed (see Skill 8-7).	
___	___	___	20. Remove gloves and dispose of them properly. Apply tie straps or tape as needed to secure the dressing.	
___	___	___	21. Return the bed to the lowest position while making the patient comfortable and raising the side rails as needed.	
___	___	___	22. Remove any remaining personal protective equipment. Remove the equipment and dispose of it properly. If any irrigating solution remains in the bottle, recap the bottle and note the date and time bottle was opened on the bottle.	
___	___	___	23. Perform hand hygiene.	
___	___	___	24. Document the procedure, wound assessment, and the patient's reaction to the according to institution's guidelines.	
___	___	___	25. Check all wound dressings every shift. You might need to check more frequently if a wound is more complex or dressings become saturated more frequently.	

Skill Checklists to Accompany Taylor's Clinical Nursing Skills:
A Nursing Process Approach

Name _____   Date _____

Unit _____   Position _____

Instructor/Evaluator: _____   Position _____

SKILL 8-10
Applying a Wound Vacuum-assisted Closure

Goal: To accomplish wound vacuum-assisted closure therapy without contaminating the wound area, causing trauma to the wound, or causing patient pain or discomfort.

Excellent	Satisfactory	Needs Practice		Comments
____	____	____	1. Review the physician's order for the application of wound vacuum-assisted closure therapy, including the ordered setting for the negative pressure.	
____	____	____	2. Gather the necessary supplies.	
____	____	____	3. Identify the patient and explain the procedure. Determine if there are allergies to any of the materials or solutions needed for the procedure.	
____	____	____	4. Perform hand hygiene.	
____	____	____	5. Close the room door or curtains. Place the bed at a comfortable working height.	
____	____	____	6. Assist the patient to a comfortable position that provides easy access to the wound area. Position him or her so the irrigation solution will flow from the upper end of the wound toward the lower end. Expose the area and drape the patient with a bath blanket if needed. Put a waterproof pad under the wound area to protect the bed.	
____	____	____	7. Have the disposal bag or waste receptacle within easy reach for use during the procedure.	
____	____	____	8. Assemble the vacuum-assisted closure device according to the manufacturer's instructions. Set the negative pressure according to the doctor's order (25 to 200 mm Hg).	
____	____	____	9. Using sterile technique, prepare a sterile field and add all the sterile supplies needed for the procedure to the field. Pour warmed sterile irrigating solution into the sterile container.	
____	____	____	10. Put on a gown, mask, and eye protection.	
____	____	____	11. Put on clean disposable gloves and remove the soiled dressings.	
____	____	____	12. Assess the wound for appearance and drainage. Assess the appearance of the surrounding tissue.	
____	____	____	13. Discard the dressings in the receptacle Remove your gloves and put them in the receptacle.	

Excellent	Satisfactory	Needs Practice		Comments
			SKILL 8-10 **Applying a Wound Vacuum-assisted** **Closure** (Continued)	
——	——	——	14. Using sterile technique, irrigate the wound as previously discussed (see Skill 8-9).	
——	——	——	15. Clean the area around the skin with normal saline. Dry the surrounding skin with a sterile gauze sponge.	
——	——	——	16. Wipe intact skin around the wound with a skin protectant; wipe and allow it to dry well.	
——	——	——	17. Remove gloves if they become contaminated and discard into the receptacle.	
——	——	——	18. Put on a new pair of sterile gloves. Using sterile scissors, cut the foam to the shape and measurement of the wound. More than one piece of foam may be necessary if the first piece is cut too small. Carefully place the foam in the wound.	
——	——	——	19. Place the fenestrated tubing into the center of the foam. There should be foam between the tubing and the base of the wound and foam over top of the tubing.	
——	——	——	20. Cover the foam and tubing with the transparent occlusive air-permeable dressing, leaving at least a 2-inch margin onto the intact skin around the wound.	
——	——	——	21. Remove and discard gloves. Connect the free end of the fenestrated tubing to the tubing that is connected to the evacuation canister.	
——	——	——	22. Turn on the vacuum unit. Observe the shrinking of the transparent dressing to the foam and skin.	
——	——	——	23. Lower the bed and make sure the patient is comfortable.	
——	——	——	24. Perform hand hygiene.	
——	——	——	25. Dispose of used supplies and equipment according to facility policy.	
——	——	——	26. Document the procedure, the pressure setting, wound assessment, and the patient's reaction according to institution's guidelines.	
——	——	——	27. Check all wound dressings every shift.	

Skill Checklists to Accompany Taylor's Clinical Nursing Skills:
A Nursing Process Approach

Name _____ Date _____

Unit _____ Position _____

Instructor/Evaluator: _____ Position _____

Excellent	Satisfactory	Needs Practice	SKILL 8-11 **Applying an External Heating Device**	Comments
			Goal: To promote wound healing and facilitate comfort through vasodilation and improved blood flow.	
___	___	___	1. Review the physician's order for the application of heat therapy, including frequency, type of therapy, body area to be treated, and length of time for the application.	
___	___	___	2. Gather the necessary supplies.	
___	___	___	3. Identify the patient and explain the procedure.	
___	___	___	4. Assess the condition of the skin where the heat is to be applied.	
___	___	___	5. Perform hand hygiene.	
___	___	___	6. Close the room door or curtains. Place the bed at a comfortable working height.	
___	___	___	7. Assist the patient to a comfortable position that provides easy access to the area to be treated. Expose the area and drape the patient with a bath blanket if needed. Put a waterproof pad under the wound area to protect the bed, if necessary.	
			For Aquathermia Pad	
___	___	___	8. Check that the water is at the appropriate level. Fill the control unit two-thirds full with distilled water or to the fill mark; if necessary, check the temperature setting on the unit to ensure it is within the safe range.	
___	___	___	9. Check for leaks and tilt the unit in several directions.	
___	___	___	10. Plug in unit and warm the pad before use. Cover the pad with an absorbent cloth. Apply the heat source to the prescribed area. Secure with gauze bandage or tape.	
___	___	___	11. Assess the condition of the skin and the patient's response to the heat at frequent intervals, according to facility policy. Do not exceed the prescribed length of time for the application of heat.	
___	___	___	12. Remove after the prescribed amount of time. Perform hand hygiene.	
___	___	___	13. Document the procedure, the patient's response, and your assessment of the area before and after application.	

*Skill Checklists to Accompany Taylor's Clinical Nursing Skills:
A Nursing Process Approach*

Name _____   Date _____

Unit _____   Position _____

Instructor/Evaluator: _____   Position _____

SKILL 8-12

Applying Warm Sterile Compresses to an Open Wound

Excellent	Satisfactory	Needs Practice	**Goal:** To promote wound healing, improve circulation, and reduce edema while keeping patient free of injury.	Comments
___	___	___	1. Review the physician's order.	
___	___	___	2. Gather the necessary supplies.	
___	___	___	3. Identify the patient and explain the procedure. Determine whether there are allergies to any of the materials or solutions needed for the procedure.	
___	___	___	4. Perform hand hygiene.	
___	___	___	5. Close the room door or curtains. Place the bed at a comfortable working height.	
___	___	___	6. Assist the patient to a comfortable position that provides easy access to the wound area. Expose the area and drape the patient with a bath blanket if needed. Put a waterproof pad under the wound area to protect the bed.	
___	___	___	7. Have a disposal bag or waste receptacle within easy reach for use during the procedure.	
___	___	___	8. Prepare any external heating pad or Aquathermia if one is being used.	
___	___	___	9. Using sterile technique, prepare a working field, open all sterile packaging, dressings, and the warmed solution. Pour the solution into the sterile container and drop the sterile gauze for compress into the solution.	
___	___	___	10. Put on clean disposable gloves and remove any old dressing in place. Discard the old dressing in the appropriate receptacle. Remove your gloves and discard as well.	
___	___	___	11. Assess wound site and surrounding tissues. Look for the presence of inflammation, drainage, skin color, ecchymosis, and odor.	
___	___	___	12. Put on sterile gloves following proper procedure.	
___	___	___	13. Retrieve sterile compress from the warmed solution, taking care to squeeze out any excess moisture from the compress. Apply the compress by gently and carefully molding the compress around the wound site.	
___	___	___	14. Cover the site with a single layer of gauze and with a dry bath towel; secure in place if necessary.	

Applying Warm Sterile Compresses
to an Open Wound *(Continued)*

Excellent	Satisfactory	Needs Practice		Comments

			15. Place any Aquathermia or heating device over the towel.	
			16. Remove your sterile gloves and discard appropriately. Perform hand hygiene.	
			17. Monitor the time the compress is in place to prevent burns or skin damage. Monitor the condition of the patient's skin and their response at frequent intervals.	
			18. After completion of the prescribed time for the treatment (up to 30 minutes), remove any external heating device and put on sterile gloves.	
			19. Carefully remove the compress while assessing the skin condition around the wound site and observing the patient's response to the heat application. Note any wound changes.	
			20. Apply a new sterile dressing to the wound following proper procedure.	
			21. Remove gloves, and place the patient in a comfortable position. Lower the bed. Dispose of any other supplies appropriately.	
			22. Perform hand hygiene.	
			23. Document the procedure, the length of time the compress was applied, your wound and surrounding tissue assessments, and the patient's response to the procedure.	

Skill Checklists to Accompany Taylor's Clinical Nursing Skills:
A Nursing Process Approach

Name _____   Date _____

Unit _____   Position _____

Instructor/Evaluator: _____   Position _____

SKILL 8-13
Using a Cooling Blanket

Goal: To maintain a normal patient body temperature without causing harm to the patient.

Excellent	Satisfactory	Needs Practice		Comments
____	____	____	1. Review the physician's order for the application of the hypothermia blanket. Obtain consent for the therapy per facility policy.	
____	____	____	2. Gather the necessary supplies.	
____	____	____	3. Identify the patient and explain the procedure.	
____	____	____	4. Assess the patient's vital signs, neurologic status, mental status, peripheral circulation, and skin integrity.	
____	____	____	5. Perform hand hygiene.	
____	____	____	6. Close the room door or curtains. Place the bed at a comfortable working height.	
____	____	____	7. Make sure the patient's gown has cloth ties, not snaps or pins.	
____	____	____	8. Apply lanolin or a mixture of lanolin and cold cream to the patient's skin where it will be in contact with the blanket.	
____	____	____	9. Turn on the blanket and make sure the cooling light is on. Verify that the pad temperature limits are set at the desired safety ranges.	
____	____	____	10. Cover the hypothermia blanket with a thin sheet or bath blanket.	
____	____	____	11. Position the blanket under the patient, so that the top edge of the pad aligns with his or her neck.	
____	____	____	12. Put on gloves. Lubricate the rectal probe and insert into the client's rectum unless contraindicated. Alternately, tuck the skin probe deep into the patient's axilla and tape it in place. For patients who are comatose or anesthetized, use an esophageal probe. Attach the probe to the control panel for the blanket.	
____	____	____	13. Wrap the patient's hands and feet in gauze if ordered or if the patient desires. For male patients, elevate scrotum off the cooling blanket with towels.	
____	____	____	14. Recheck the thermometer and settings on the control panel.	

Excellent	Satisfactory	Needs Practice		Comments
			SKILL 8-13 **Using a Cooling Blanket** *(Continued)*	
___ ___ ___			15. Remove gloves and perform hand hygiene.	
___ ___ ___			16. Turn and position the patient regularly, every 30 minutes to 1 hour. Keep linens free from condensation. Reapply cream as needed. Observe the patient's skin for indications of change in color, changes in lips and nailbeds, edema, pain, and sensory impairment.	
___ ___ ___			17. Monitor the patient's vital signs and perform a neurologic assessment per facility policy, usually every 15 minutes until the body temperature is stable.	
___ ___ ___			18. Observe for signs of shivering, including verbalized sensations, facial muscle twitching, hyperventilation, or twitching of extremities.	
___ ___ ___			19. Assess the patient's level of comfort.	
___ ___ ___			20. Turn off blanket according to facility policy, usually when the patient's body temperature reaches 1 degree above the desired temperature. Continue to monitor the patient's temperature until it stabilizes.	
___ ___ ___			21. Document assessments, vital signs, and time of initiation of therapy. Document the control settings, the duration of treatment, and patient responses.	

Skill Checklists to Accompany Taylor's Clinical Nursing Skills:
A Nursing Process Approach

Name _____   Date _____

Unit _____   Position _____

Instructor/Evaluator: _____   Position _____

SKILL 8-14

Applying Cold Therapy

Goal: To assist the patient to experience increased comfort, decreased muscle spasms, or decreased inflammation without showing signs of bleeding or hematoma at the treatment site.

Excellent	Satisfactory	Needs Practice		Comments
___	___	___	1. Review the physician's order for the application of cold therapy, including frequency, type of therapy, body area to be treated, and length of time for the application.	
___	___	___	2. Gather the necessary supplies.	
___	___	___	3. Identify the patient and explain the procedure.	
___	___	___	4. Assess the condition of the skin where the ice is to be applied.	
___	___	___	5. Perform hand hygiene.	
___	___	___	6. Close the room door or curtains. Place the bed at a comfortable working height.	
___	___	___	7. Assist the patient to a comfortable position that provides easy access to the area to be treated. Expose the area and drape the patient with a bath blanket if needed. Put a waterproof pad under the wound area to protect the bed, if necessary.	
___	___	___	8. Fill the bag, collar, or glove about three-fourths full with ice. Remove any excess air from the device. Securely fasten the end of the bag or collar; tie the glove closed.	
___	___	___	9. Cover the device with the towel or washcloth. If the device has a cloth exterior, this is not necessary.	
___	___	___	10. Put on gloves. Remove and dispose of any dressings at the site, if present.	
___	___	___	11. Place the device lightly against the area. Remove the ice and assess the site for redness after 30 seconds. Ask the patient about the presence of burning sensations.	
___	___	___	12. Replace the device snugly against the site if no problems are evident. Secure in place with gauze wrap or tape.	
___	___	___	13. Reassess the treatment area every 5 minutes or according to facility policy.	
___	___	___	14. After 20 minutes or the prescribed amount of time, remove the ice and dry the skin.	
___	___	___	15. Apply a new dressing to site, if necessary.	
___	___	___	16. Perform hand hygiene.	
___	___	___	17. Document the procedure, the patient's response, and your assessment of the area before and after application.	

Skill Checklists to Accompany Taylor's Clinical Nursing Skills:
A Nursing Process Approach

Name _____ Date _____

Unit _____ Position _____

Instructor/Evaluator: _____ Position _____

Excellent	Satisfactory	Needs Practice	SKILL 8-15 **Applying Montgomery Straps**	Comments
			Goal: To keep the patient's skin free from irritation and injury; Montgomery straps are applied without contaminating the wound area, causing trauma to the wound, or causing patient pain or discomfort.	
____	____	____	1. Review the physician's order for wound care or the nursing care plan related to wound care.	
____	____	____	2. Gather the necessary supplies.	
____	____	____	3. Identify the patient. Explain the procedure to the patient. Inquire about any known allergies, specifically related to the products being used for wound care.	
____	____	____	4. Perform hand hygiene.	
____	____	____	5. Close the room door or curtains. Place the bed at an appropriate and comfortable working height.	
____	____	____	6. Place a waste receptacle at a convenient location for use during the procedure.	
____	____	____	7. Assist the patient to a comfortable position that provides easy access to the wound area. Use a bath blanket to cover any exposed area other than the wound. If necessary, place a waterproof pad under the wound site.	
____	____	____	8. Perform wound care and a dressing change as outlined in Skill 8-7, as ordered.	
____	____	____	9. If ready-made straps are not available, cut four to six strips of tape, long enough to extend about 6 inches beyond the wound. The number of strips will depend of the size of the wound and dressing.	
____	____	____	10. Fold one of each strip 2 to 3 inches back on itself, sticky sides together, to form a nonadhesive tab. Cut a small hole in the folded tab's center, close to the top edge. Make as many pairs of straps as necessary to secure the dressing.	
____	____	____	11. Put on clean gloves. Clean the patient's skin on either side of the wound with the gauze, moistened with normal saline. Dry the skin.	

Excellent	Satisfactory	Needs Practice	SKILL 8-15 **Applying Montgomery Straps** *(Continued)*	Comments
——	——	——	12. Apply a skin protectant to the skin where the straps will be placed.	
——	——	——	13. Remove gloves.	
——	——	——	14. Apply the sticky side of each tape or strap to a skin barrier sheet. Apply the sheet directly to the skin near the dressing. Repeat for the other side.	
——	——	——	15. Thread a separate string through each pair of holes in the straps. Tie one end of the string in the hole. Fasten the other end with the opposing tie, like a shoelace. Do not secure too tightly. Repeat according to the number of straps needed. If commercially prepared straps are used, tie strings like a shoelace. Note date and time of application on strap.	
——	——	——	16. Return the bed to the lowest position while making the patient comfortable and raising the side rails as needed.	
——	——	——	17. Perform hand hygiene.	
——	——	——	18. Document the procedure, the patient's response, and your assessment of the area before and after application.	
——	——	——	19. Replace the ties and straps whenever they are soiled or every 2 to 3 days.	

Name _____   Date _____

Unit _____   Position _____

Instructor/Evaluator: _____   Position _____

SKILL 8-16
Applying a Saline-Moistened Dressing

Excellent	Satisfactory	Needs Practice		Comments
			Goal: To accomplish the procedure without contaminating the wound area, causing trauma to the wound, or causing the patient to experience pain or discomfort; and to maintain sterile technique if appropriate.	
____	____	____	1. Review the physician's order and/or nursing care plan for the application of a saline-moistened dressing.	
____	____	____	2. Gather the necessary supplies.	
____	____	____	3. Identify the patient and explain the procedure. Determine if the patient is allergic to any of the materials or solutions needed for the procedure.	
____	____	____	4. Perform hand hygiene.	
____	____	____	5. Close the room door or curtains. Place the bed at a comfortable working height.	
____	____	____	6. Assist the patient to a comfortable position that provides easy access to the wound area. Position the patient so the irrigation solution will flow from the upper end of the wound toward the lower end, if wound irrigation is necessary. Expose the area and drape the patient with the bath blanket if needed. Put the waterproof pad under the wound area to protect the bed.	
____	____	____	7. Have the disposal bag or waste receptacle within easy reach.	
____	____	____	8. Put on personal protective equipment as appropriate.	
____	____	____	9. Put on clean disposable gloves and gently remove the soiled dressings. If the dressing adheres to the underlying tissues, moisten it with saline to loosen.	
____	____	____	10. After removing the dressing, note the presence, amount, type, color, and odor of any drainage on the dressings. Place soiled dressings in the appropriate waste receptacle.	
____	____	____	11. Assess the wound for appearance, stage, the presence of eschar, granulation tissue, epithelialization, undermining, tunneling, necrosis, sinus tract, and drainage. Assess the appearance of the surrounding tissue. Measure the wound.	
____	____	____	12. Remove your gloves and put them in the receptacle.	

Excellent	Satisfactory	Needs Practice	SKILL 8-16 **Applying a Saline-Moistened Dressing** *(Continued)*	
				Comments
___	___	___	13. Using sterile technique, open the supplies and dressings. Place the fine-mesh gauze into the basin and pour the ordered solution over the mesh to saturate it.	
___	___	___	14. Put on the sterile gloves.	
___	___	___	15. Cleanse or irrigate the wound as prescribed or with normal saline. (See Skills 8-7 and 8-9.)	
___	___	___	16. Apply a skin protectant to the skin surrounding the wound.	
___	___	___	17. Squeeze excess fluid from the gauze dressing. Unfold and fluff the dressing.	
___	___	___	18. Gently press the moistened gauze into the wound. If necessary, use the forceps or cotton-tipped applicators to press the gauze into all wound surfaces.	
___	___	___	19. Apply several dry, sterile gauze pads over the wet gauze.	
___	___	___	20. Place the ABD pad over the gauze.	
___	___	___	21. Remove and discard your sterile gloves. Apply tape or tie tapes to secure the dressings.	
___	___	___	22. After securing the dressing, remove all remaining equipment, place the patient in a position of comfort with side rails up and the bed in the lowest position, and perform hand hygiene.	
___	___	___	23. Record the procedure, your wound assessment, and the patient's reaction to the procedure using your institution's guidelines.	
___	___	___	24. Check all wound dressings every shift. You might need to check more frequently if a wound is more complex or dressings become saturated more frequently.	

Skill Checklists to Accompany Taylor's Clinical Nursing Skills:
A Nursing Process Approach

Name _____   Date _____

Unit _____   Position _____

Instructor/Evaluator: _____   Position _____

SKILL 8-17
Applying a Hydrocolloid Dressing

Goal: To accomplish the procedure without contaminating the wound area, causing trauma to the wound, or causing the patient to experience pain or discomfort; and to maintain sterile technique if appropriate.

Excellent	Satisfactory	Needs Practice		Comments
___	___	___	1. Review the physician's order and/or nursing care plan for the application of a hydrocolloid dressing.	
___	___	___	2. Gather the necessary supplies.	
___	___	___	3. Identify the patient and explain the procedure. Determine if the patient is allergic to any of the materials or solutions needed for the procedure.	
___	___	___	4. Perform hand hygiene.	
___	___	___	5. Close the room door or curtains. Place the bed at a comfortable working height.	
___	___	___	6. Assist the patient to a comfortable position that provides easy access to the wound area. Position the patient so the irrigation solution will flow from the upper end of the wound toward the lower end, if necessary. Expose the area and drape the patient with the bath blanket if needed. Put the waterproof pad under the wound area to protect the bed.	
___	___	___	7. Have the disposal bag or waste receptacle within easy reach.	
___	___	___	8. Put on personal protective equipment as appropriate.	
___	___	___	9. Put on clean disposable gloves and gently remove the soiled dressing. Discard it in the receptacle.	
___	___	___	10. Assess the wound for appearance, stage, granulation tissue, epithelialization, undermining, tunneling, necrosis, sinus tract, and drainage. Assess the appearance of the surrounding tissue. Measure the wound.	
___	___	___	11. Remove your gloves and put them in the receptacle.	
___	___	___	12. Set up a sterile field and put on the sterile gloves if indicated.	
___	___	___	13. Cleanse or irrigate the wound as prescribed or with normal saline. (See Skills 8-7 and 8-9.)	

Excellent	Satisfactory	Needs Practice	SKILL 8-17 **Applying a Hydrocolloid Dressing** *(Continued)*	
				Comments
___	___	___	14. Apply a skin protectant to the skin surrounding the wound.	
___	___	___	15. Choose a clean, dry, presized dressing or cut one to size using sterile scissors. The dressing must be sized generously, allowing at least a 1″ margin of healthy skin around the wound to be covered with the dressing.	
___	___	___	16. Remove the release paper from the adherent side of the dressing. Apply the dressing to the wound without stretching the dressing. Smooth wrinkles as it is applied.	
___	___	___	17. If necessary, secure the dressing edges with tape. Dressings that are near the anus need to have the edges taped. Apply additional skin barrier to the areas to be covered with tape, if necessary.	
___	___	___	18. Remove and discard your sterile gloves.	
___	___	___	19. Remove all remaining equipment, place the patient in a position of comfort with side rails up and the bed in the lowest position, and perform hand hygiene.	
___	___	___	20. Record the procedure, your wound assessment, and the patient's reaction to the procedure using your institution's guidelines. Note the date for the next dressing change, based on facility policy (normally 3 to 7 days).	
___	___	___	21. Check all wound dressings every shift to validate that they are intact.	

Skill Checklists to Accompany Taylor's Clinical Nursing Skills:
A Nursing Process Approach

Name _____   Date _____

Unit _____   Position _____

Instructor/Evaluator: _____   Position _____

Excellent	Satisfactory	Needs Practice	SKILL 9-1 **Assisting Patient to Turn in Bed**	Comments
			Goal: To promote patient comfort and proper body alignment without injury to the patient or nurse.	
——	——	——	1. Review the physician's orders and nursing plan of care for patient activity. Identify any movement limitations and the ability of the patient to assist with turning.	
——	——	——	2. Gather any positioning aids, if necessary.	
——	——	——	3. Identify the patient. Explain the procedure to the patient.	
——	——	——	4. Perform hand hygiene and put on gloves, if necessary.	
——	——	——	5. Close the room door or curtains. Place the bed at an appropriate and comfortable working height.	
——	——	——	6. Adjust the head of the bed to a flat position or as low as the patient can tolerate. Place pillows, wedges, or any other supports to be used for positioning within easy reach.	
——	——	——	7. Using the drawsheet, move the patient to the edge of the bed, opposite the side to which he or she will be turned.	
——	——	——	8. Stand on the side of the bed toward which the patient is turning. Make sure the side rail on the opposite side of the bed from where you are standing is raised. Lower the side rail nearest you.	
——	——	——	9. Place the patient's arms across the chest and cross his or her far leg over the leg nearest to you.	
——	——	——	10. Stand opposite the patient's center with your feet spread about shoulder width and with one foot ahead of the other. Tighten your gluteal and abdominal muscles and flex your knees. Use your leg muscles to do the pulling.	
——	——	——	11. Position your hands on the patient's far shoulder and hip and roll the patient toward you. Or, you may use the drawsheet to gently pull the patient over on his or her side.	
——	——	——	12. Use a pillow or other support behind the patient's back. Pull the shoulder blade forward and out from under the patient.	
——	——	——	13. Make the patient comfortable and position in proper alignment, using pillows or other supports under the leg	

Excellent	Satisfactory	Needs Practice	SKILL 9-1 **Assisting Patient to Turn in Bed** *(Continued)*	Comments
			and arm as needed. Readjust the pillow under his or her head. Elevate the head of the bed as needed for comfort.	
___	___	___	14. Place the bed in the lowest position, with the side rails up. Make sure the call bell and other necessary items are within easy reach.	
___	___	___	15. Perform hand hygiene and document the position change per your facility's policy.	

Name _____ Date _____

Unit _____ Position _____

Instructor/Evaluator: _____ Position _____

SKILL 9-2

Providing Range-of-Motion Exercises

Excellent	Satisfactory	Needs Practice	**Goal:** To move each joint through its range of motion to promote mobility and improve circulation.	Comments
——	——	——	1. Review the physician's orders and nursing plan of care for patient activity. Identify any movement limitations.	
——	——	——	2. Identify the patient. Explain the procedure to the patient.	
——	——	——	3. Perform hand hygiene and put on gloves, if necessary.	
——	——	——	4. Close the room door or curtains. Place the bed at an appropriate and comfortable working height. Adjust the head of the bed to a flat position or as low as the patient can tolerate.	
——	——	——	5. Stand on the side of the bed where the joints are to be exercised. Only uncover the limb to be used during the exercise.	
——	——	——	6. Perform the exercises slowly and gently, providing support by holding the areas proximal and distal to the joint. Repeat each exercise two to five times, moving each joint in a smooth and rhythmic manner. Stop movement if the patient complains of pain or if you meet resistance.	
——	——	——	7. Perform the exercises beginning at the head and moving down one side of the body at a time.	
——	——	——	8. Start at the patient's head. Move her chin down to rest on her chest. Then return her head to a normal upright position. Tilt her head as far as possible toward each shoulder.	
——	——	——	9. Next, move to her neck. Move the head from side to side, bringing her chin toward each shoulder.	
——	——	——	10. Move down to her shoulder. Start with her arm at her side and lift the arm forward to above her head. Return her arm to the starting position at the side of her body.	
——	——	——	11. With her arm back at her side, move the arm laterally to an upright position above her head, then return to the original position. Move the arm across his body as far as possible.	
——	——	——	12. Next, raise her arm at her side until her upper arm is in line with her shoulder. Bend her elbow at a 90-degree angle and move her forearm upward and downward, and then return the arm to her side.	

Excellent	Satisfactory	Needs Practice	SKILL 9-2 **Providing Range-of-Motion Exercises** (Continued)	
				Comments
___	___	___	13. Continue the exercises at the elbow. Bend the elbow and move her lower arm and hand upward toward her shoulder. Return the lower arm and hand to the original position while straightening the elbow.	
___	___	___	14. For the forearm, rotate her lower arm and hand so her palm is up. Then, rotate her lower arm and hand so the palm of her hand is down.	
___	___	___	15. Move to her wrist. Move her hand downward toward the inner aspect of her forearm. Return her hand to a neutral position even with her forearm. Then move the dorsal portion of her hand backward as far as possible.	
___	___	___	16. Continue by bending her fingers to make a fist, and then straighten them out. Spread the fingers apart and return them back together. Touch her thumb to each finger on her hand.	
___	___	___	17. Then move to the hip. Extend her leg and lift it upward. Return her leg to the original position beside the other leg.	
___	___	___	18. Then, lift her leg laterally away from her body. Return the leg back toward the other leg and try to extend beyond the midline if possible.	
___	___	___	19. Next, turn the foot and leg toward the other leg to rotate it internally. Turn the foot and leg outward away from the other leg to rotate it externally.	
___	___	___	20. Move to her knee. Bend her leg and bring the heel toward the back of her leg, and then return the leg to a straight position.	
___	___	___	21. At the ankle, move her foot up and back until her toes are upright. Move her foot with her toes pointing downward.	
___	___	___	22. Then, turn the sole of her foot toward the midline. Turn the sole of her foot outward.	
___	___	___	23. Curl her toes downward, then straighten them out. Spread the toes apart and bring them together.	
___	___	___	24. Repeat these exercises with the other side of her body. Remember to encourage the patient to do as many of these exercises by herself as possible.	
___	___	___	25. When finished, make sure the patient is comfortable, with the side rails up and bed in the lowest position.	
___	___	___	26. Remove gloves if used and perform hand hygiene. Document the exercises performed, any observations, and the patient's reaction to the activities.	

Skill Checklists to Accompany Taylor's Clinical Nursing Skills:
A Nursing Process Approach

Name _____   Date _____

Unit _____   Position _____

Instructor/Evaluator: _____   Position _____

SKILL 9-3
Moving a Patient Up in Bed with the Assistance of Another Nurse

Goal: To promote comfort, improve circulation, and maintain proper body alignment while keeping patient free from injury.

Excellent	Satisfactory	Needs Practice		Comments
——	——	——	1. Review the medical record and nursing plan of care for conditions that may influence the patient's ability to move or to be positioned. Assess for tubes, intravenous lines, incisions, or equipment that may alter the positioning procedure. Identify any movement limitations.	
——	——	——	2. Identify the patient. Explain the procedure to the patient.	
——	——	——	3. Perform hand hygiene and put on gloves, if necessary.	
——	——	——	4. Close the room door or curtains. Place the bed at an appropriate and comfortable working height. Adjust the head of the bed to a flat position or as low as the patient can tolerate.	
——	——	——	5. Remove all pillows from under the patient. Leave one at the head of the bed, leaning upright against the headboard.	
——	——	——	6. Position one nurse on either side of the bed and lower both side rails.	
——	——	——	7. If a drawsheet is not in place under the patient, take a moment to place one under the patient's midsection.	
——	——	——	8. If patient is able, ask the patient to bend his legs and put his feet flat on the bed to assist with the movement.	
——	——	——	9. Have the patient fold his arms across his chest. If able, have him lift his head with his chin on his chest.	
——	——	——	10. Position yourself at the patient's midsection with your feet spread shoulder width apart and one foot slightly in front of the other.	
——	——	——	11. Fold or bunch the drawsheet close to the patient before grasping it securely and preparing to move the patient.	
——	——	——	12. Flex knees and hips. Tighten abdominal and gluteal muscles and keep your back straight.	
——	——	——	13. Shift your weight back and forth from your back leg to your front leg and count to three. On the count of three, move the patient up in bed. If possible, the patient can assist the move by pushing with his legs. Repeat the	

SKILL 9-3

Moving a Patient Up in Bed with the Assistance of Another Nurse *(Continued)*

Excellent	Satisfactory	Needs Practice		Comments
			process if necessary to get the patient to the right position.	
—	—	—	14. Assist the patient to a comfortable position and readjust the pillows and supports as needed. Raise the side rails. Place the bed in the lowest position.	
—	—	—	15. Perform hand hygiene.	

Skill Checklists to Accompany Taylor's Clinical Nursing Skills:
A Nursing Process Approach

Name _____   Date _____

Unit _____   Position _____

Instructor/Evaluator: _____   Position _____

Excellent	Satisfactory	Needs Practice	SKILL 9-4 **Transferring a Patient from the Bed to a Stretcher**	Comments
			Goal: To promote safety and prevent patient and nurse injury.	
___	___	___	1. Review the medical record and nursing plan of care for conditions that may influence the patient's ability to move or to be positioned. Assess for tubes, intravenous lines, incisions, or equipment that may alter the positioning procedure. Identify any movement limitations.	
___	___	___	2. Identify the patient. Explain the procedure to the patient.	
___	___	___	3. Perform hand hygiene and put on gloves, if necessary.	
___	___	___	4. Close the room door or curtains. Adjust the head of the bed to a flat position or as low as the patient can tolerate. Raise the bed to the same height as the transport stretcher. Lower the side rails.	
___	___	___	5. Place a drawsheet under the patient if one is not already there. Have patient fold arms across chest and move chin to chest. Use the drawsheet to move the patient to the side of the bed where the stretcher will be placed.	
___	___	___	6. Place a bath blanket over the patient and remove the top covers from underneath.	
___	___	___	7. Position the stretcher next to and parallel to the bed. Lock the wheels on the stretcher and the bed.	
___	___	___	8. Remove the pillow from the bed and place it on the stretcher. The two nurses should stand on the stretcher side of the bed. The third nurse should stand on the side of the bed without the stretcher.	
___	___	___	9. Have the nurse on the side of the bed without the stretcher kneel on the bed, with his or her knee at the upper torso closer to the patient than the other knee. Fold or bunch the drawsheet close to the patient before grasping it securely in preparation for the transfer.	
___	___	___	10. Have one of the nurses on the stretcher side of the bed reach across the stretcher and grasp the drawsheet at the head and chest areas of the patient.	
___	___	___	11. Have the other nurse reach across the stretcher and grasp the drawsheet at the patient's waist and thigh area.	

Excellent	Satisfactory	Needs Practice	SKILL 9-4 **Transferring a Patient from the Bed to a Stretcher** *(Continued)*	
				Comments
___	___	___	12. At a signal given by one of the nurses, have the nurses standing on the stretcher side of the bed pull the sheet. At the same time, the nurse kneeling on the bed should lift the patient from the bed to the stretcher.	
___	___	___	13. Once the patient is transferred to the stretcher, secure the patient until the side rails are raised. Raise the side rails. Ensure the patient's comfort. Cover with a blanket. Leave the drawsheet in place for the return transfer.	
___	___	___	14. Perform hand hygiene and document the time and patient's destination, according to facility policy.	

Skill Checklists to Accompany Taylor's Clinical Nursing Skills:
A Nursing Process Approach

Name _____   Date _____

Unit _____   Position _____

Instructor/Evaluator: _____   Position _____

Excellent	Satisfactory	Needs Practice	SKILL 9-5 **Transferring a Patient from the Bed to a Chair** **Goal:** To promote safety, prevent injury to patient and nurse, and maintain body alignment.	Comments
___	___	___	1. Review the medical record and nursing plan of care for conditions that may influence the patient's ability to move or to be positioned. Assess for tubes, intravenous lines, incisions, or equipment that may alter the positioning procedure. Identify any movement limitations.	
___	___	___	2. Identify the patient. Explain the procedure to the patient.	
___	___	___	3. Perform hand hygiene and put on gloves, if necessary.	
___	___	___	4. If needed, move the equipment to make room for the chair. Close the door or draw the curtains.	
___	___	___	5. Place the bed in the lowest position. Raise the head of the bed to a sitting position or as high as the patient can tolerate.	
___	___	___	6. Make sure the bed brakes are locked. Put the chair right next to the bed, facing the foot of the bed. If the chair does not have brakes, brace the chair against a secure object. Whenever available, lock the brakes of the chair.	
___	___	___	7. Assist the patient to a side-lying position, facing the side of the bed the patient will sit on. Lower the side rail if necessary, and stand near the patient's hips. Stand with your legs shoulder width apart with one foot near the head of the bed, slightly in front of the other foot.	
___	___	___	8. Ask the patient to swing her legs over the side of the bed. At the same time, pivot on your back leg to lift the patient's trunk and shoulders. Remember to keep your back straight, avoid twisting.	
___	___	___	9. Stand in front of the patient and assess for any balance problems or complaints of dizziness. Allow legs to dangle a few minutes before continuing.	
___	___	___	10. Assist the patient to put on a robe and nonskid footwear.	
___	___	___	11. Stand facing the patient. Spread your feet about shoulder width and flex your hips and knees.	
___	___	___	12. Place your hands around the patient's waist while the patient holds on to you with one hand on your shoulder	

Excellent	Satisfactory	Needs Practice		Comments
			SKILL 9-5 **Transferring a Patient from the Bed to a Chair** (*Continued*)	

Excellent	Satisfactory	Needs Practice		Comments
			and the other hand on your waist. Apply a transfer belt if necessary.	
___	___	___	13. Ask the patient to slide buttocks to the edge of the bed, until her feet touch the floor. Position yourself as close to patient as possible with one foot positioned on the outside of the patient's foot.	
___	___	___	14. Rock back and forth while counting to three. On the count of three, use your legs (not your back) to help raise the patient to a standing position. If indicated, brace your front knee against the patient's weak extremity as she stands.	
___	___	___	15. Pivot on your back foot until the patient feels the chair against her legs.	
___	___	___	16. Ask the patient to use her arm to steady herself on the arm of the chair while slowly lowering to a sitting position. Continue to brace her knees with your knees. Flex your hips and knees when helping her sit in the chair.	
___	___	___	17. Assess the patient's alignment in the chair. Cover with a blanket if needed. Place the call bell close so it is available for use.	
___	___	___	18. Perform hand hygiene. Document the activity, including the length of time the patient sat in the chair, any observations, and the patient's tolerance and reaction to the activity.	

Skill Checklists to Accompany Taylor's Clinical Nursing Skills:
A Nursing Process Approach

Name _____   Date _____

Unit _____   Position _____

Instructor/Evaluator: _____   Position _____

SKILL 9-6

Transferring a Patient from a Bed to a Chair with the Assistance of Another Nurse

Goal: To promote safety, prevent injury, and maintain body alignment for a patient requiring total assistance.

Excellent	Satisfactory	Needs Practice		Comments
___	___	___	1. Review the medical record and nursing plan of care for conditions that may influence the patient's ability to move or to be positioned. Assess for tubes, intravenous lines, incisions, or equipment that may alter the positioning procedure. Identify any movement limitations.	
___	___	___	2. Identify the patient. Explain the procedure to the patient.	
___	___	___	3. Perform hand hygiene and put on gloves, if necessary.	
___	___	___	4. If needed, move the equipment to make room for the chair. Close the door or draw the curtains.	
___	___	___	5. Make sure the bed brakes are locked. Adjust the height of the bed to comfortable working height or at the level of the armrest (if one is present) on the chair.	
___	___	___	6. Move the patient to the near side of the bed while patient crosses his arms on his chest if possible. Position the chair next to the bed near the upper end and with the back of the chair parallel to the head of the bed. If possible, remove the armrest closest to the bed. Lock the chair wheels, if available. Use a chair transfer board if appropriate.	
___	___	___	7. Prepare to lift the patient from the bed to the chair. Have the lead nurse stand behind the chair and slip his or her arms under the patient's axillae and grasp the patient's wrists securely. The second nurse faces the wheelchair and supports the patient's knees by placing his or her arms under the patient's knees.	
___	___	___	8. On a predetermined signal, flex hips and knees, keeping backs straight and simultaneously lifting the patient and gently lowering patient into the chair. If necessary, use a chair transfer board.	
___	___	___	9. Adjust the patient's position using pillows if necessary. Check his alignment in the chair. Cover the patient with a blanket if necessary. Place the call bell within reach.	
___	___	___	10. Perform hand hygiene. Document the activity, transfer, any observations, the patient's tolerance, and the length of time in the chair.	

128

Skill Checklists to Accompany Taylor's Clinical Nursing Skills:
A Nursing Process Approach

Name _____   Date _____

Unit _____   Position _____

Instructor/Evaluator: _____   Position _____

Excellent	Satisfactory	Needs Practice	SKILL 9-7 **Transferring a Patient Using a Hydraulic Lift**	Comments
			Goal: To transfer the patient without injury to the patient or nurse and promote mobility.	
___	___	___	1. Review the medical record and nursing plan of care for conditions that may influence the patient's ability to move or to be positioned. Assess for tubes, intravenous lines, incisions, or equipment that may alter the positioning procedure. Identify any movement limitations.	
___	___	___	2. Identify the patient. Explain the procedure to the patient.	
___	___	___	3. Perform hand hygiene and put on gloves, if necessary.	
___	___	___	4. If needed, move the equipment to make room for the chair. Close the door or draw the curtains.	
___	___	___	5. Bring the chair to the side of the bed. Lock the wheels, if present.	
___	___	___	6. Adjust the bed to a comfortable working height. Lock the bed brakes.	
___	___	___	7. Place the sling evenly under the patient. Roll the patient to one side and place half of the sling with the sheet or pad on it under the patient from shoulders to midthigh. Roll the patient to the other side and pull the sling under the patient.	
___	___	___	8. Roll the base of the lift under the side of the bed nearest to the chair. Center the frame over the patient. Lock the wheels of the lift.	
___	___	___	9. Using the base-adjustment lever, widen the stance of the base.	
___	___	___	10. Lower the arms close enough to attach the sling to the frame.	
___	___	___	11. Place the strap or chain hooks through the holes of the sling. Short straps attach behind the patient's back and long straps at the other end. Check the patient to make sure the hooks are not pressing into the skin. Some lifts have straps on the sling that attach to hooks on the frame. Check the manufacturer's instructions for the specifics for each particular lift.	
___	___	___	12. Check all equipment, lines, and drains attached to the patient so that they are not interfering with the device.	

Excellent	Satisfactory	Needs Practice		Comments
			Instruct the patient to fold his or her arms across the chest.	
___	___	___	13. With a person standing on each side of the lift, tell the patient that he or she will be lifted from the bed. Support injured limbs as necessary. Engage the pump to raise the patient about 6 inches above the bed.	
___	___	___	14. Unlock the wheels of the lift. Carefully wheel the patient straight back and away from the bed. Support the patient's limbs as needed.	
___	___	___	15. Position the patient over the chair with the base of the lift straddling the chair. Lock the wheels of the lift.	
___	___	___	16. Gently lower the patient to the chair until the hooks or straps are slightly loosened from the sling or frame. Guide the patient into the chair with your hands as the sling lowers.	
___	___	___	17. Disconnect the hooks or strap from the frame. Keep the sling in place under the patient.	
___	___	___	18. Adjust the patient's position using pillows if necessary. Check his or her alignment in the chair. Cover the patient with a blanket if necessary. Place the call bell within reach. When time for the patient to return to bed, reattach the hooks or straps and reverse the steps.	
___	___	___	19. Perform hand hygiene. Document the activity, transfer, any observations, the patient's tolerance of the procedure, and the length of time in the chair.	

130

Skill Checklists to Accompany Taylor's Clinical Nursing Skills:
A Nursing Process Approach

Name _____   Date _____

Unit _____   Position _____

Instructor/Evaluator: _____   Position _____

Excellent	Satisfactory	Needs Practice	SKILL 9-8 **Assisting a Patient with Ambulation** **Goal:** To ambulate the patient safely without experiencing falls or injury.	Comments
___	___	___	1. Review the medical record and nursing plan of care for conditions that may influence the patient's ability to move and ambulate. Assess for tubes, intravenous lines, incisions, or equipment that may alter the procedure for ambulation. Identify any movement limitations.	
___	___	___	2. Identify the patient. Explain the procedure to the patient. Explain that the patient is to report any feelings of dizziness, weakness, or shortness of breath while walking. Decide how far to walk.	
___	___	___	3. Perform hand hygiene.	
___	___	___	4. Place the bed in the lowest position.	
___	___	___	5. Assist the patient to the side of the bed. Have the patient sit on the side of the bed for several minutes and assess for dizziness or lightheadedness. Have the patient stay sitting until he or she feels secure.	
___	___	___	6. Assist the patient with footwear and a robe, if desired.	
___	___	___	7. Wrap the transfer belt around the patient waist, based on assessed need and facility policy.	
___	___	___	8. Assist the patient to stand. Have the patient hold your waist or shoulders for support when standing, if needed. Assess the patient's balance and leg strength. If the patient is weak or unsteady, return the patient to bed or assist to a chair.	
___	___	___	9. When one nurse assists, position yourself to the side and slightly behind the patient. Support the patient by the waist or transfer belt.	
___	___	___	a. When two nurses assist, position yourself to the side and slightly behind the patient, supporting the patient by the waist or transfer belt. Have the other nurse carry or manage equipment or provide additional support from the other side.	
___	___	___	b. Alternatively, when two nurses assist, stand at the patient's sides (one nurse on each side) with near hands grasping the inferior aspect of the patient's near upper	

Assisting a Patient with Ambulation *(Continued)*

Excellent	Satisfactory	Needs Practice		Comments
			arm and far hands holding the patient's lower arm or hand.	
___	___	___	c. Or possibly, when two nurses assist, stand at the patient's sides (one nurse on each side), slip near arms under the patient's arms and around his or her back, grasping each other's arms. Have the patient stretch his or her arms over the nurses' shoulders and then grasp the patient's hands with your far hands.	
___	___	___	10. Take several steps forward with the patient. Continue to assess patient strength and balance. Remind patient to stand erect.	
___	___	___	11. Continue with ambulation for the planned distance and time. Return the patient to the bed or chair based on the patient's tolerance and condition.	
___	___	___	12. Perform hand hygiene. Document the activity, any observations, the patient's tolerance of the procedure, and the distance walked.	

Name _____ Date _____

Unit _____ Position _____

Instructor/Evaluator: _____ Position _____

Excellent	Satisfactory	Needs Practice	SKILL 9-9 **Assisting a Patient with Ambulation Using a Walker** **Goal:** To assist patient to ambulate safely with a walker and be free from falls or injury.	Comments
____	____	____	1. Review the medical record and nursing plan of care for conditions that may influence the patient's ability to move and ambulate and for specific instructions for ambulation, such as distance. Assess for tubes, intravenous lines, incisions, or equipment that may alter the procedure for ambulation. Assess the patient's knowledge and previous experience regarding the use of a walker. Identify any movement limitations.	
____	____	____	2. Identify the patient. Explain the procedure to the patient. Encourage the patient to report any feelings of dizziness, weakness, or shortness of breath while walking. Decide how far to walk.	
____	____	____	3. Perform hand hygiene.	
____	____	____	4. Place the bed in the lowest position.	
____	____	____	5. Assist the patient to the side of the bed. Have the patient sit on the side of the bed. Assess for dizziness or lightheadedness. Have the patient stay sitting until he feels secure. Alternatively, assist patient to chair.	
____	____	____	6. Assist the patient with footwear and a robe, if desired.	
____	____	____	7. Place the walker directly in front of the patient. Ask the patient to push himself off the bed, or assist patient to stand if seated in a chair. Assist the patient to stand within the walker, if necessary. Once standing, have the patient hold the handgrips firmly and equally, while standing slightly behind, on one side.	
____	____	____	8. Have the patient move the walker forward 6 to 8 inches and set it down, making sure all four feet of the walker stay on the floor. Then, tell patient to step forward with either foot into the walker, supporting himself on his arms. Follow through with the other leg. If one leg is weaker or impaired, have patient step forward with the involved leg and follow with the uninvolved leg, again supporting himself on his arms.	
____	____	____	9. Move the walker forward again and continue the same pattern. Continue with ambulation for the planned	

Excellent	Satisfactory	Needs Practice	SKILL 9-9 **Assisting a Patient with Ambulation Using a Walker** *(Continued)*	
				Comments
			distance and time. Return the patient to the bed or chair based on patient tolerance.	
___	___	___	10. Perform hand hygiene. Document the activity, any observations, the patient's ability to use the walker, the patient's tolerance of the procedure, and the distance walked.	

134

Name _____ Date _____

Unit _____ Position _____

Instructor/Evaluator: _____ Position _____

Excellent	Satisfactory	Needs Practice	SKILL 9-10 **Assisting a Patient with Ambulation Using Crutches** **Goal:** To assist a patient to ambulate safely without experiencing falls or injury.	Comments
___	___	___	1. Review the medical record and nursing plan care for conditions that may influence the patient's ability to move and ambulate. Assess for tubes, intravenous lines, incisions, or equipment that may alter the procedure for ambulation. Assess the patient's knowledge and previous experience regarding the use of crutches. Determine that the appropriate size crutch has been obtained.	
___	___	___	2. Identify the patient. Explain the procedure to the patient. Explain that the patient is to report any feelings of dizziness, weakness, or shortness of breath while walking. Decide how far to walk.	
___	___	___	3. Perform hand hygiene.	
___	___	___	4. Assist the patient to stand erect, face forward in the tripod position. This means the patient holds the crutches 6 inches in front of and 6 inches to the side of each foot.	
___	___	___	5. For the four-point gait,	
___	___	___	a. Have the patient move the right crutch forward 6 inches and then move left foot forward to the level of the right crutch.	
___	___	___	b. Then have the patient move the left crutch forward 6 inches and then move the right foot forward to the level of the left crutch.	
___	___	___	6. For the three-point gait,	
___	___	___	a. Have the patient move the affected leg and both crutches forward about 6 inches.	
___	___	___	b. Have the patient move the stronger leg forward to the level of the crutches.	
___	___	___	7. For the two-point gait,	
___	___	___	a. Have the patient move the left crutch and the right foot forward about 6 inches at the same time.	
___	___	___	b. Have the patient move the right crutch and left leg forward to the level of the left crutch at the same time.	

Assisting a Patient with
Ambulation Using Crutches *(Continued)*

Excellent	Satisfactory	Needs Practice		Comments
——	——	——	8. For the swing-to gait,	
——	——	——	a. Have the patient move both crutches forward about 6 inches.	
——	——	——	b. Have the patient lift his legs and swing them to the crutches, supporting his body weight on the crutches.	
——	——	——	9. For the swing-through gait,	
——	——	——	a. Have the patient move both crutches forward about 6 inches.	
——	——	——	b. Have the patient lift his legs and swing through and ahead of the crutches, supporting his weight on the crutches.	
——	——	——	10. Continue with ambulation for the planned distance and time. Return the patient to the bed or chair based on the patient's tolerance and condition.	
——	——	——	11. Perform hand hygiene. Document the activity, any observations, the patient's ability to use the crutches, the patient's tolerance of the procedure, and the distance walked.	

Skill Checklists to Accompany Taylor's Clinical Nursing Skills:
A Nursing Process Approach

Name _____ Date _____

Unit _____ Position _____

Instructor/Evaluator: _____ Position _____

Excellent	Satisfactory	Needs Practice	SKILL 9-11 **Assisting a Patient with Ambulation Using a Cane**	
			Goal: To assist a patient to ambulate safely without experiencing falls or injury.	**Comments**
____	____	____	1. Review the medical record and nursing plan of care for conditions that may influence the patient's ability to move and ambulate. Assess for tubes, intravenous lines, incisions, or equipment that may alter the procedure for ambulation. Assess the patient's knowledge and previous experience regarding the use of a cane. Identify any movement limitations.	
____	____	____	2. Identify the patient. Explain the procedure to the patient. Explain that the patient is to report any feelings of dizziness, weakness, or shortness of breath while walking. Decide how far to walk.	
____	____	____	3. Perform hand hygiene.	
____	____	____	4. Assist the patient to stand with weight evenly distributed between the feet and the cane.	
____	____	____	5. Have the patient hold the cane on the patient's stronger side, close to his body.	
____	____	____	6. Tell the patient to advance the cane 4 to 12 inches (10 to 30 cm) and then, while supporting his weight on the stronger leg and the cane, advance the weaker foot forward, parallel with the cane.	
____	____	____	7. While supporting weight on the weaker leg and the cane, have the patient advance the stronger leg forward ahead of the cane (heel slightly beyond the tip of the cane).	
____	____	____	8. Tell the patient to move the weaker leg forward until even with the stronger leg and then advance the cane again.	
____	____	____	9. Continue with ambulation for the planned distance and time. Return the patient to the bed or chair based on the patient's tolerance and condition.	
____	____	____	10. Perform hand hygiene. Document the activity, any observations, the patient's ability to use the cane, the patient's tolerance of the procedure, and the distance walked.	

Skill Checklists to Accompany Taylor's Clinical Nursing Skills:
A Nursing Process Approach

Name _____   Date _____

Unit _____   Position _____

Instructor/Evaluator: _____   Position _____

Excellent	Satisfactory	Needs Practice	SKILL 9-12 **Applying Pneumatic Compression Devices**	Comments
			Goal: To promote adequate circulation in the extremities of the patient; patient is without symptoms of neurovascular compromise.	
____	____	____	1. Review the medical record and nursing plan of care for conditions that may contraindicate the use of the compression device.	
____	____	____	2. Identify the patient. Explain the procedure to the patient.	
____	____	____	3. Perform hand hygiene.	
____	____	____	4. Close the room door or curtains. Place the bed at an appropriate and comfortable working height.	
____	____	____	5. Hang the compression pump on the foot of the patient's bed and plug it into an electrical outlet. Attach the connecting tubing to the pump.	
____	____	____	6. Remove the compression sleeves from the package and unfold them. Lay the unfolded sleeves on the bed with the cotton lining facing up. Take note of the markings indicating the correct placement for the ankle and popliteal areas.	
____	____	____	7. Place a sleeve under the patient's leg with the tubing toward his or her heel. Each one fits either leg. For total leg sleeves, place the behind-the-knee opening at the popliteal space to prevent pressure there. For knee-high sleeves, make sure the back of the ankle is over the ankle marking.	
____	____	____	8. Wrap the sleeve snugly around the patient's leg so that two fingers fit between the leg and the sleeve. Secure the sleeve with the Velcro fasteners. Repeat for the second leg, if bilateral therapy is ordered. Connect each sleeve to the tubing for the pump. Follow the manufacturer's recommendations for connecting.	
____	____	____	9. Set the pump to the prescribed maximum pressure. The usual maximum pressure setting is 35 to 55 mm Hg. Make sure the tubing is free from kinks and that the patient can turn about without interrupting the airflow. Turn on the pump.	
____	____	____	10. Observe the patient and the device for the first cycle of the device. Check the audible alarms. Check the sleeves and pump at least once per shift or per facility policy.	

Excellent	Satisfactory	Needs Practice	SKILL 9-12 **Applying Pneumatic Compression Devices** *(Continued)*	Comments
——	——	——	11. Place the bed in the lowest position, with the side rails up. Make sure the call bell and other necessary items are within easy reach.	
——	——	——	12. Assess the extremities for peripheral pulses, edema, changes in sensation, and movement. Remove the sleeves and assess and document skin integrity every 8 hours.	
——	——	——	13. Perform hand hygiene. Document the time and date of application of the pneumatic compression device, the patient's response to the therapy, and their understanding of the therapy. Document the status of the alarms and the cooling settings.	

Skill Checklists to Accompany Taylor's Clinical Nursing Skills:
A Nursing Process Approach

Name _____   Date _____

Unit _____   Position _____

Instructor/Evaluator: _____   Position _____

SKILL 9-13
Applying a Continuous Passive Motion Device

Excellent	Satisfactory	Needs Practice	**Goal:** To promote increased joint mobility.	Comments
___	___	___	1. Review the medical record and nursing plan of care for the appropriate degrees of flexion and extension, the cycle rate, and the length of time for use of the continuous passive motion (CPM) device.	
___	___	___	2. Identify the patient. Explain the procedure to the patient.	
___	___	___	3. Obtain equipment. Apply the soft goods to the CPM device.	
___	___	___	4. Perform hand hygiene.	
___	___	___	5. Close the room door or curtains. Place the bed at an appropriate and comfortable working height.	
___	___	___	6. Using the tape measure, determine the distance between the gluteal crease and the popliteal space.	
___	___	___	7. Measure the length of the patient's leg from the knee to ¼ inch beyond the bottom of the foot.	
___	___	___	8. Position the patient in the middle of the bed. The affected extremity should be in a slightly abducted position.	
___	___	___	9. Support the affected extremity and elevate it, placing it in the padded CPM device.	
___	___	___	10. Check to make sure the patient's knee is at the hinged joint of the CPM device.	
___	___	___	11. Adjust the footplate to maintain the patient's foot in a neutral position. Check to make sure the leg is not internally or externally rotated.	
___	___	___	12. Apply the restraining straps under the CPM device and around the leg. Check that two fingers fit between the strap and the leg.	
___	___	___	13. Explain the use of the STOP/GO button to the patient. Set the controls to the levels ordered by the physician. Turn on the power to the CPM device.	
___	___	___	14. Set the device to ON and start the therapy by pressing the GO button. Observe the patient and the device for the first cycle of the device. Determine the angle of flexion when the device reaches its greatest height using the goniometer.	

Excellent	Satisfactory	Needs Practice	

SKILL 9-13
Applying a Continuous Passive Motion Device
(Continued)

Comments

Excellent	Satisfactory	Needs Practice		Comments
___	___	___	15. Check the patient's level of comfort and perform skin and neurovascular assessment at least every 8 hours or per facility policy.	
___	___	___	16. Place the bed in the lowest position, with the side rails up. Make sure the call bell and other necessary items are within easy reach.	
___	___	___	17. Perform hand hygiene. Document the time and date of application of the CPM device, the extension and flexion settings, the speed of the device, the patient's response to the therapy, and your assessment of the extremity.	

Skill Checklists to Accompany Taylor's Clinical Nursing Skills:
A Nursing Process Approach

Name _____   Date _____

Unit _____   Position _____

Instructor/Evaluator: _____   Position _____

Excellent	Satisfactory	Needs Practice	SKILL 9-14 **Applying a Sling**	Comments
			Goal: To assist the patient to maintain muscle strength and joint range of motion.	
___	___	___	1. Review the medical record and nursing plan of care to determine the need for the use of a sling.	
___	___	___	2. Identify the patient. Explain the procedure to the patient.	
___	___	___	3. Perform hand hygiene.	
___	___	___	4. Close the room door or curtains. Place the bed at an appropriate and comfortable working height, if necessary.	
___	___	___	5. Assist the patient to a sitting position. Place the patient's forearm across the chest with the elbow flexed and the palm against the chest. Measure the sleeve length, if indicated.	
___	___	___	6. Enclose the arm in the sling, making sure the elbow fits into the corner of the fabric. Run the strap up the patient's back and across the shoulder opposite the injury, and then down the chest to the fastener on the end of the sling.	
___	___	___	7. Place the ABD pad under the strap, between the strap and the patient's neck. Ensure the sling and forearm are slightly elevated and at a right angle to the body.	
___	___	___	8. Place the bed in the lowest position, with the side rails up. Make sure the call bell and other necessary items are within easy reach.	
___	___	___	9. Check the patient's level of comfort, arm positioning, and neurovascular status of the affected limb every 4 hours or according to facility policy. Assess the axillary and cervical skin frequently for irritation or breakdown.	
___	___	___	10. Perform hand hygiene. Document the time and date that the sling was applied. Document the patient's response to the sling and the neurovascular status of the extremity.	

Skill Checklists to Accompany Taylor's Clinical Nursing Skills:
A Nursing Process Approach

Name _____   Date _____

Unit _____   Position _____

Instructor/Evaluator: _____   Position _____

Excellent	Satisfactory	Needs Practice	SKILL 9-15 **Applying a Figure-of-Eight Bandage** **Goal:** To assist patient to maintain circulation to the affected part and remain free of neurovascular complications.	Comments
___	___	___	1. Review the medical record and nursing plan of care to determine the need for the use of a figure-of-eight bandage.	
___	___	___	2. Identify the patient. Explain the procedure to the patient.	
___	___	___	3. Perform hand hygiene and put on gloves if contact with drainage is possible.	
___	___	___	4. Close the room door or curtains. Place the bed at an appropriate and comfortable working height.	
___	___	___	5. Assist the patient to a comfortable position, with the affected body part in a normal functioning position.	
___	___	___	6. Hold the bandage roll with the roll facing upward in one hand. Hold the free end of the roll in the other hand. Hold the bandage so it is close to the affected body part.	
___	___	___	7. Wrap the bandage around the limb twice, below the joint, in place, to anchor it.	
___	___	___	8. Use alternating ascending and descending turns to form a figure eight. Overlap each turn of the bandage by one-half to two-thirds the width of the strip.	
___	___	___	9. Unroll the bandage as you wrap. Do not unroll the entire bandage before wrapping.	
___	___	___	10. Wrap firmly, but not tightly. Assess the patient's comfort as you wrap. If the patient reports tingling, itching, numbness, or pain, loosen the bandage.	
___	___	___	11. After area is covered, wrap the bandage around the limb twice, above the joint, in place, to anchor it. Secure the end of the bandage with tape, pins, or self-closures. Avoid metal clips.	
___	___	___	12. Remove your gloves, if worn, and discard. Place the bed in the lowest position, with the side rails up. Make sure the call bell and other necessary items are within easy reach.	
___	___	___	13. Assess the distal circulation after the bandage is in place.	
___	___	___	14. Elevate a wrapped extremity for 15 to 30 minutes after application of the bandage.	

Excellent	Satisfactory	Needs Practice	SKILL 9-15 **Applying a Figure-of-Eight Bandage** *(Continued)*	Comments
___	___	___	15. Lift the distal end of the bandage and assess the skin for color, temperature, and integrity. Assess for pain and perform a neurovascular assessment for the affected extremity at least every 4 hours or per facility policy.	
___	___	___	16. Remove and change the bandage at least once a day or per physician order or facility policy. Cleanse the skin and dry thoroughly before applying a new bandage. Assess the skin for irritation and breakdown.	
___	___	___	17. Perform hand hygiene. Document the time, date, and site that the bandage was applied and the size bandage used. Include the skin assessment and care provided before application. Document the patient's response to the bandage and the neurovascular status of the extremity.	

Skill Checklists to Accompany Taylor's Clinical Nursing Skills:
A Nursing Process Approach

Name _____ Date _____

Unit _____ Position _____

Instructor/Evaluator: _____ Position _____

SKILL 9-16

Assisting with Cast Application

Goal: To assist with applying a cast that does not interfere with neurovascular function and healing.

Excellent	Satisfactory	Needs Practice		Comments
——	——	——	1. Review the medical record and physician's orders to determine the need for the application of a cast.	
——	——	——	2. Identify the patient. Explain the procedure to the patient and verify area to be casted.	
——	——	——	3. Perform a pain assessment, including assessing for muscle spasm. Administer prescribed medications in sufficient time to allow for the full effect of the analgesic and/or muscle relaxant.	
——	——	——	4. Perform hand hygiene and put on gloves, if necessary.	
——	——	——	5. Close the room door or curtains. Place the bed at an appropriate and comfortable working height, if necessary.	
——	——	——	6. Position the patient as needed, depending on the type of cast being applied and the location of the injury. Support the extremity or body part to be casted.	
——	——	——	7. Drape the patient with waterproof pads.	
——	——	——	8. Cleanse and dry the affected body part.	
——	——	——	9. Position and maintain the affected body part in the position indicated by the physician as the stockinette, sheet wadding, and padding is applied. The stockinette should extend beyond the ends of the cast. As the wadding is applied, check for wrinkles.	
——	——	——	10. Position and maintain the affected body part in the position indicated by the physician as the casting material is applied. Assist with finishing by folding the stockinette or other padding down over the outer edge of the cast.	
——	——	——	11. Support the cast during hardening. Handle hardening plaster casts with the palms of hands, not fingers. Support the cast on a firm smooth surface. Do not rest on hard surface or sharp edges. Avoid pressure on the cast.	
——	——	——	12. Elevate the injured limb above heart level with pillow or bath blankets as ordered, making sure pressure is evenly distributed under the cast.	

Assisting with Cast Application *(Continued)*

Excellent	Satisfactory	Needs Practice		Comments
——	——	——	13. Remove gloves and dispose of them properly; place the bed in the lowest position, if necessary.	
——	——	——	14. Obtain x-rays as ordered.	
——	——	——	15. Instruct the patient to report pain, odor, drainage, changes in sensation, abnormal sensation, or the inability to move fingers or toes of the affected extremity.	
——	——	——	16. Leave the cast uncovered and exposed to the air. Reposition the patient every 2 hours. Depending on facility policy, a fan may be used to dry the cast.	
——	——	——	17. Perform hand hygiene. Document the time, date, and site to which the cast was applied. Include the skin assessment and care provided before application. Document the patient's response to the cast and the neurovascular status of the extremity.	

146

Skill Checklists to Accompany Taylor's Clinical Nursing Skills:
A Nursing Process Approach

Name _____   Date _____

Unit _____   Position _____

Instructor/Evaluator: _____   Position _____

<table>
<tr><th>Excellent</th><th>Satisfactory</th><th>Needs Practice</th><th>SKILL 9-17
Caring for a Cast

Goal: To ensure that the cast remains intact without causing neurovascular compromise.</th><th>Comments</th></tr>
<tr><td>____</td><td>____</td><td>____</td><td>1. Review the medical record and the nursing plan of care to determine the need for cast care and care for the affected body part.</td><td></td></tr>
<tr><td>____</td><td>____</td><td>____</td><td>2. Identify the patient. Explain the procedure to the patient.</td><td></td></tr>
<tr><td>____</td><td>____</td><td>____</td><td>3. Perform hand hygiene and put on gloves, if necessary.</td><td></td></tr>
<tr><td>____</td><td>____</td><td>____</td><td>4. Close the room door or curtains. Place the bed at an appropriate and comfortable working height, if necessary.</td><td></td></tr>
<tr><td>____</td><td>____</td><td>____</td><td>5. If a plaster cast was applied, handle the casted extremity or body area with the palms of your hands for the first 24 to 36 hours until the cast is fully dry.</td><td></td></tr>
<tr><td>____</td><td>____</td><td>____</td><td>6. If the cast is on an extremity, elevate the affected area on pillows covered with waterproof pads. Maintain the normal curvatures and angles of the cast.</td><td></td></tr>
<tr><td>____</td><td>____</td><td>____</td><td>7. Keep cast (plaster) uncovered until fully dry.</td><td></td></tr>
<tr><td>____</td><td>____</td><td>____</td><td>8. Wash excess antiseptic or antimicrobial agents, such as povidone iodine (Betadine), or residual casting material from the exposed skin. Dry thoroughly.</td><td></td></tr>
<tr><td>____</td><td>____</td><td>____</td><td>9. Assess the condition of the cast. Be alert for cracks, dents, or the presence of drainage from the cast. Perform skin and neurovascular assessment according to facility policy, as often as every 1 to 2 hours. Check for pain, edema, inability to move body parts distal to the cast, pallor, pulses, and the presence of abnormal sensations. If the cast is on an extremity, compare with the uncasted extremity.</td><td></td></tr>
<tr><td>____</td><td>____</td><td>____</td><td>10. If breakthrough bleeding or drainage is noted on the cast, mark the area on the cast. Indicate the date and time next to the area. Follow physician orders or facility policy regarding the amount of drainage that needs to be reported to the physician.</td><td></td></tr>
<tr><td>____</td><td>____</td><td>____</td><td>11. Assess for signs of infection. Monitor the patient's temperature, the presence of foul odor from the cast, increased pain, or extreme warmth over an area of the cast.</td><td></td></tr>
</table>

Excellent	Satisfactory	Needs Practice	SKILL 9-17 **Caring for a Cast** *(Continued)*	Comments
——	——	——	12. Reposition the patient every 2 hours. Provide back and skin care frequently. Encourage range of motion for unaffected joints. Encourage the patient to cough and breathe deeply.	
——	——	——	13. Instruct the patient to report pain, odor, drainage, changes in sensation, abnormal sensation, or the inability to move fingers or toes of the affected extremity.	
——	——	——	14. Remove gloves and dispose of them appropriately; place the bed in the lowest position, if necessary.	
——	——	——	15. Perform hand hygiene. Document all assessments and care provided. Document the patient's response to the cast, repositioning, and any teaching.	

Skill Checklists to Accompany Taylor's Clinical Nursing Skills:
A Nursing Process Approach

Name _____   Date _____

Unit _____   Position _____

Instructor/Evaluator: _____   Position _____

SKILL 9-18
Applying Skin Traction and Caring for a Patient in Skin Traction

Goal: To apply skin traction maintained with the appropriate counterbalance, keeping the patient free from complications of immobility.

Excellent	Satisfactory	Needs Practice		Comments
___	___	___	1. Review the medical record and the nursing plan of care to determine the type of traction being used and care for the affected body part.	
___	___	___	2. Identify the patient. Explain the procedure to the patient, emphasizing the importance of maintaining counterbalance, alignment, and position.	
___	___	___	3. Perform a pain assessment, including assessing for muscle spasm. Administer prescribed medications in sufficient time to allow for the full effect of the analgesic and/or muscle relaxant.	
___	___	___	4. Perform hand hygiene.	
___	___	___	5. Close the room door or curtains. Place the bed at an appropriate and comfortable working height.	
___	___	___	6. Ensure the traction apparatus is attached securely to the bed. Assess the traction setup. Apply the ordered amount of weight. The weights should hang freely, not touching the bed or the floor.	
___	___	___	7. Check that the ropes move freely through the pulleys. Check that all knots are tight and are positioned away from the pulleys. Pulleys should be free from the linens.	
___	___	___	8. Place the patient in a supine position with the foot of the bed elevated slightly. The patient's head should be near the head of the bed and in alignment.	
___	___	___	9. Cleanse the affected area. Place the elastic hose on the affected limb.	
___	___	___	10. Place the traction boot over the patient's leg. Be sure the patient's heel is in the heel of the boot. Secure the boot with the straps.	
___	___	___	11. Attach the traction cord to the footplate of the boot. Pass the rope over the pulley fastened at the end of the bed. Attach the weight to the hook on the rope, usually 5 to 10 pounds for an adult. Gently let go of the weight.	

Excellent	Satisfactory	Needs Practice		Comments
——	——	——	12. Check the patient's alignment with the traction.	
——	——	——	13. Perform a skin traction assessment per facility policy. This assessment includes checking the traction equipment, examining the affected body part, maintaining proper body alignment, and performing a skin assessment and a neurovascular assessment.	
——	——	——	14. Check the boot for placement and alignment. Make sure the line of pull is parallel to the bed and not angled downward.	
——	——	——	15. Remove the straps every 4 hours per physician's order or facility policy. Check bony prominences for skin breakdown, abrasions, and pressure areas. Remove the boot per physician's order or facility policy every 8 hours. Put on gloves and wash, rinse, and thoroughly dry the skin.	
——	——	——	16. Assess the extremity distal to the traction for edema and the status of peripheral pulses. Assess the temperature, color, and capillary refill and compare with the unaffected limb. Check for pain, inability to move body parts distal to the traction, pallor, and the presence of abnormal sensations. Assess for indicators of deep vein thrombosis, including calf tenderness, swelling, and a positive Homans sign.	
——	——	——	17. Replace the traction and remove gloves and dispose of appropriately.	
——	——	——	18. Ensure the patient is positioned in the center of the bed with the affected leg aligned with the trunk of his or her body.	
——	——	——	19. Periodically examine the weights and pulley system. Weights should hang freely, off the floor and bed. Knots should be secure. Ropes should move freely through the pulleys. The pulleys should not be constrained by knots.	
——	——	——	20. Perform range-of-motion exercises on all joint areas, unless contraindicated. Encourage the patient to cough and breathe deeply every 2 hours.	
——	——	——	21. Raise the side rails. Place the bed in the lowest position that still allows the weight to hang freely.	
——	——	——	22. Perform hand hygiene. Document the time, date, type, amount of weight used, and the site that the traction was applied. Include the skin assessment and care provided before application. Document the patient's response to the traction and the neurovascular status of the extremity.	

Skill Checklists to Accompany Taylor's Clinical Nursing Skills:
A Nursing Process Approach

Name _____   Date _____

Unit _____   Position _____

Instructor/Evaluator: _____   Position _____

SKILL 9-19
Caring for a Patient in Skeletal Traction

Goal: To maintain traction appropriately, keeping the patient free from the complications of immobility and infection.

Excellent	Satisfactory	Needs Practice		Comments
___	___	___	1. Review the medical record and the nursing plan of care to determine the type of traction being used and the prescribed care.	
___	___	___	2. Identify the patient. Explain the procedure to the patient, emphasizing the importance of maintaining counterbalance, alignment, and position.	
___	___	___	3. Perform a pain assessment, including assessing for muscle spasm. Administer prescribed medications in sufficient time to allow for the full effect of the analgesic and/or muscle relaxant.	
___	___	___	4. Perform hand hygiene.	
___	___	___	5. Close the room door or curtains. Place the bed at an appropriate and comfortable working height.	
___	___	___	6. Ensure the traction apparatus is attached securely to the bed. Assess the traction setup, including application of the ordered amount of weight. Be sure that the weights hang freely, not touching the bed or the floor.	
___	___	___	7. Check that the ropes move freely through the pulleys. Check that all knots are tight and are positioned away from the pulleys. Pulleys should be free from the linens.	
___	___	___	8. Check the alignment of the patient's body as prescribed.	
___	___	___	9. Perform a skin assessment. Pay attention to pressure points, including the ischial tuberosity, popliteal space, Achilles tendon, sacrum, and heel.	
___	___	___	10. Perform a neurovascular assessment. Assess the extremity distal to the traction for edema and the status of peripheral pulses. Assess the temperature and color and compare with the unaffected limb. Check for pain, inability to move body parts distal to the traction, pallor, and the presence of abnormal sensations. Assess for indicators of deep vein thrombosis, including calf tenderness, swelling, and a positive Homans sign.	
___	___	___	11. Assess the site at and around the pins for redness, edema, and odor. Assess for skin tenting, prolonged or purulent	

SKILL 9-19

Caring for a Patient in Skeletal Traction *(Continued)*

Excellent	Satisfactory	Needs Practice		Comments
			drainage, elevated body temperature, elevated pin-site temperature, and bowing or bending of the pins.	
___	___	___	12. Provide pin-site care.	
___	___	___	a. Using sterile technique, open the applicator package and pour the cleansing agent into the sterile container.	
___	___	___	b. Put on the sterile gloves.	
___	___	___	c. Place the applicators into the solution.	
___	___	___	d. Clean the pin site, starting at the insertion area and working outward, away from the pin site.	
___	___	___	e. Use each applicator once. Use a new applicator for each pin site.	
___	___	___	13. Depending on physician order and facility policy, apply the antimicrobial ointment to pin sites and apply a dressing.	
___	___	___	14. Perform range-of-motion exercises on all joint areas, unless contraindicated. Encourage the patient to cough and breathe deeply every 2 hours.	
___	___	___	15. Remove gloves. Perform hand hygiene. Document the time, date, type of traction, and the amount of weight used. Include the skin assessment, pin-site assessment, and pin-site care. Document the patient's response to the traction and the neurovascular status of the extremity.	

Name _____   Date _____

Unit _____   Position _____

Instructor/Evaluator: _____   Position _____

SKILL 9-20

Caring for a Patient with an External Fixation Device

Goal: To ensure patient shows no evidence of complications when using an external fixation device.

Excellent	Satisfactory	Needs Practice		Comments
___	___	___	1. Review the medical record and the nursing plan of care to determine the type of device being used and prescribed care.	
___	___	___	2. Identify the patient. Explain the procedure to the patient. Assure the patient that there will be little pain after the fixation device is in place. Reinforce that he or she will be able to adjust to the device. Reinforce the fact that he or she will be able to move about with the device, allowing normal activities to be resumed more quickly.	
___	___	___	3. After the fixation device is in place, apply ice to the surgical site as ordered or per facility policy. Elevate the affected body part, if appropriate.	
___	___	___	4. Perform a pain assessment, including assessing for muscle spasm. Administer prescribed medications in sufficient time to allow for the full effect of the analgesic and/or muscle relaxant.	
___	___	___	5. Administer analgesics as ordered before exercising or mobilizing the affected body part.	
___	___	___	6. Perform neurovascular assessments per facility policy or physician's order, usually every 2 to 4 hours for 24 hours and then every 4 to 8 hours. Assess the affected body part for color, motion, sensation, edema, capillary refill, and pulses. If appropriate, compare with the unaffected side. Assess for pain not relieved by analgesics, burning, tingling, and numbness.	
___	___	___	7. Perform hand hygiene.	
___	___	___	8. Close the room door or curtains. Place the bed at an appropriate and comfortable working height.	
___	___	___	9. Assess the pin site for redness, tenting of the skin, prolonged or purulent drainage, swelling, and bowing, bending, or loosening of the pins. Monitor body temperature.	
___	___	___	10. Perform pin-site care.	
___	___	___	a. Using sterile technique, open the applicator package and pour the cleansing agent into the sterile container.	

Caring for a Patient with an External Fixation Device *(Continued)*

Excellent	Satisfactory	Needs Practice		Comments

Excellent	Satisfactory	Needs Practice		Comments
___	___	___	b. Put on the sterile gloves.	
___	___	___	c. Place the applicators into the solution.	
___	___	___	d. Clean the pin site, starting at the insertion area and working outward, away from the pin site.	
___	___	___	e. Use each applicator once. Use a new applicator for each pin site.	
___	___	___	11. Depending on physician order and facility policy, apply the antimicrobial ointment to pin sites and apply a dressing.	
___	___	___	12. Remove gloves. Perform hand hygiene. Document the time, date, and type of device in place. Include the skin assessment, pin-site assessment, and pin-site care. Document the patient's response to the device and the neurovascular status of the affected area.	

Skill Checklists to Accompany Taylor's Clinical Nursing Skills:
A Nursing Process Approach

Name _____   Date _____

Unit _____   Position _____

Instructor/Evaluator: _____   Position _____

Excellent	Satisfactory	Needs Practice	SKILL 9-21 **Caring for a Patient in Halo Traction** **Goal:** To maintain cervical alignment.	Comments
___	___	___	1. Review the medical record and the nursing plan of care to determine the type of device being used and prescribed care.	
___	___	___	2. Identify the patient. Explain the procedure to the patient.	
___	___	___	3. Perform hand hygiene.	
___	___	___	4. Close the room door or curtains. Place the bed at a comfortable working height, or have patient sit up if appropriate.	
___	___	___	5. Monitor vital signs and perform a neurologic assessment, including level of consciousness, motor function, and sensation, per facility policy. This is usually at least every 2 hours for 24 hours or possibly every hour for 48 hours.	
___	___	___	6. Examine the halo vest unit every 8 hours for stability, secure connections, and position. Check to make sure that the patient's head is centered in the halo without neck flexion or extension. Check each bolt for loosening.	
___	___	___	7. Check the fit of the vest. With the patient in a supine position, you should be able to insert one or two fingers under the jacket at the shoulder and chest.	
___	___	___	8. Wash the patient's chest and back daily. Place the patient on his or her back or sitting upright if appropriate. Loosen the bottom Velcro straps.	
___	___	___	9. Wring out a bath towel soaked in warm water. Pull the towel back and forth in a drying motion beneath the front. Do not use soap or lotion under the vest.	
___	___	___	10. Thoroughly dry the skin in the same manner with a dry towel. Inspect the skin for tender reddened areas or pressure spots. Lightly dust the skin with a prescribed medicated powder or cornstarch.	
___	___	___	11. Turn the patient on his or her side less than 45 degrees if lying supine and repeat the process on his or her back. Close the Velcro straps. Assist the patient with changing the shirt.	

Excellent	Satisfactory	Needs Practice	SKILL 9-21 **Caring for a Patient in Halo Traction** *(Continued)*	
				Comments
——	——	——	12. Perform a respiratory assessment. Check for respiratory impairment, such as absence of breath sounds, the presence of adventitious sounds, reduced inspiratory effort, or the presence of shortness of breath.	
——	——	——	13. Assess the pin site for redness, tenting of the skin, prolonged or purulent drainage, swelling, and bowing, bending, or loosening of the pins. Monitor body temperature.	
——	——	——	14. Perform pin-site care (see Skills 9-19 and 9-20).	
——	——	——	15. Depending on physician order and facility policy, apply the antimicrobial ointment to pin sites and apply a dressing.	
——	——	——	16. Remove gloves and dispose of appropriately. Place the bed in the lowest position.	
——	——	——	17. Perform hand hygiene. Document the time, date, and type of device in place. Include the skin assessment, pin-site assessment, and pin-site care. Document the patient's response to the device and the neurologic and respiratory assessment.	

Skill Checklists to Accompany Taylor's Clinical Nursing Skills:
A Nursing Process Approach

Name _____   Date _____

Unit _____   Position _____

Instructor/Evaluator: _____   Position _____

SKILL 10-1

Giving a Back Massage

			Goal: To promote comfort and relaxation.	**Comments**

Excellent	Satisfactory	Needs Practice		
___	___	___	1. Explain the procedure and offer back massage to patient.	
___	___	___	2. Perform hand hygiene.	
___	___	___	3. Close curtain or door.	
___	___	___	4. Assist patient to the prone position or side-lying position with the back exposed from the shoulders to the sacral area. Use a bath blanket to drape patient. Raise bed to the highest position and lower side rail closest to you.	
___	___	___	5. Warm lubricant or lotion in your palm or place container in warm water.	
___	___	___	6. Using light gliding strokes (effleurage), apply lotion to patient's shoulders, back, and sacral area.	
___	___	___	7. Place your hands beside each other at the base of patient's spine and stroke upward to shoulders and back and downward to buttocks in slow continuous strokes. Continue for several minutes, applying additional lotion as necessary.	
___	___	___	8. Massage patient's shoulders, entire back, areas over iliac crests, and sacrum with circular stroking motion. Keep your hands in contact with patient's skin. Continue for several minutes, applying additional lotion as necessary.	
___	___	___	9. Knead patient's skin by gently alternating grasping and compression motions (pétrissage).	
___	___	___	10. Complete massage with additional long stroking movements that eventually become lighter in pressure with movement of fingertips downward.	
___	___	___	11. During massage, observe patient's skin for reddened or open areas. Pay particular attention to skin over bony prominences.	
___	___	___	12. Use a towel to pat patient dry and to remove excess lotion. Apply powder if patient requests it.	
___	___	___	13. Perform hand hygiene.	
___	___	___	14. Assess patient's response and record your observations on patient's chart.	

Skill Checklists to Accompany Taylor's Clinical Nursing Skills:
A Nursing Process Approach

Name _____   Date _____

Unit _____   Position _____

Instructor/Evaluator: _____   Position _____

Excellent	Satisfactory	Needs Practice	SKILL 10-2 **Applying a TENS Unit**	Comments
			Goal: To decrease pain without the patient experiencing injury of skin irritation or breakdown.	
___	___	___	1. Identify the patient, show the patient the device, and explain the function of the device and reason for use.	
___	___	___	2. Perform hand hygiene.	
___	___	___	3. Inspect the area where the electrodes are to be placed. Clean and dry it with an alcohol wipe.	
___	___	___	4. Remove the adhesive backing from the electrodes and apply to the specified location. If the electrodes are not pre-gelled, apply a small amount of electrode gel to the bottom of each electrode. If not self-adhering, tape the electrodes in place.	
___	___	___	5. Check the placement to ensure leaving at least a 2-inch (5-cm) space (about the width of one electrode) between them.	
___	___	___	6. Note the controls on the TENS unit to make sure they are off. Connect the wires to the electrodes (if not already attached) and plug them into the unit.	
___	___	___	7. Turn on the unit and adjust the intensity setting to the lowest intensity and determine whether the patient can feel a tingling, burning, or buzzing sensation. Then adjust the intensity to the prescribed amount or the setting most comfortable for the patient. Secure the unit to the patient.	
___	___	___	8. Set the pulse width (duration of the each pulsation) as indicated or recommended.	
___	___	___	9. Assess the patient's pain during therapy.	
			a. If intermittent use is ordered, turn the unit off after the specified duration of treatment and remove the electrodes. Provide skin care to the area.	
___	___	___	b. If continuous therapy is ordered, periodically remove the electrodes from the skin (after turning the unit off) to inspect the area and clean the skin. Reapply electrodes and continue therapy.	
___	___	___	10. When therapy is discontinued, turn the unit off and remove the electrodes. Clean the patient's skin. Clean the unit and replace the batteries.	

Excellent	Satisfactory	Needs Practice	SKILL 10-2 **Applying a TENS Unit** *(Continued)*	
				Comments
——	——	——	11. Perform hand hygiene and document the date and time of application, patient's initial pain assessment, electrode placement location, intensity and pulse width, duration of therapy, pain assessments during therapy and patient's response, and time of removal or discontinuation of therapy.	

Skill Checklists to Accompany Taylor's Clinical Nursing Skills:
A Nursing Process Approach

Name _____   Date _____

Unit _____   Position _____

Instructor/Evaluator: _____   Position _____

Excellent	Satisfactory	Needs Practice	SKILL 10-3 **Caring for a Patient Receiving PCA**	
			Goal: To decrease pain as verbalized by the patient.	**Comments**
___	___	___	1. Identify the patient, show the patient the device, and explain the function of the device and reason for use.	
___	___	___	2. Plug the patient-controlled analgesia (PCA) device into the electrical outlet.	
___	___	___	3. Perform hand hygiene and put on gloves.	
___	___	___	4. Check the label on the prefilled drug syringe with the medication record and patient identification.	
___	___	___	5. Connect tubing to prefilled syringe and place the syringe into the PCA device. Prime the tubing.	
___	___	___	6. Connect the PCA tubing to the patient's intravenous infusion line or subcutaneous infusion port; tape the connection site.	
___	___	___	7. Set the PCA device to administer the loading dose and then program the device based on the physician's order for infusion dosage and lock-out interval.	
___	___	___	8. Instruct the patient to press the button each time he or she needs relief from pain.	
___	___	___	9. Continue to assess the patient's pain at least every 1 to 2 hours and monitor vital signs, especially respiratory status. Inspect site of infusion and rate periodically. Replace the drug syringe when empty.	
___	___	___	10. Remove gloves and dispose of them appropriately and perform hand hygiene. Document the date and time of initiating PCA therapy, initial pain assessment, drug and loading dose administered, individual dosing and time interval, continued pain assessments, and patient's response to therapy.	

Skill Checklists to Accompany Taylor's Clinical Nursing Skills:
A Nursing Process Approach

Name _____   Date _____

Unit _____   Position _____

Instructor/Evaluator: _____   Position _____

Excellent	Satisfactory	Needs Practice	SKILL 10-4 **Caring for a Patient Receiving Epidural Analgesia** **Goal:** To decrease patient pain as verbalized by the patient.	Comments
____	____	____	1. Verify the physician's order for analgesia, drug preparation, and rate of infusion with another registered nurse. Perform hand hygiene and put on gloves if indicated.	
____	____	____	2. Have an ampule of 0.4 mg of naloxone (Narcan) and a syringe at the bedside.	
____	____	____	3. After the catheter has been inserted, check the infusion bag and ensure that the infusion tubing has been primed and connected to the epidural catheter and rate of infusion is correct.	
____	____	____	4. Tape all connection sites and label bag, tubing, and pump apparatus "For Epidural Infusion Only." Do not administer any other narcotics or adjuvant drugs without approval of clinician responsible for epidural injection.	
____	____	____	5. Assess the exit site and apply a transparent dressing over the catheter insertion site. Monitor infusion rate.	
____	____	____	6. Assess and record sedation level (using a sedation scale) and respiratory status every hour for the first 24 hours followed by every 4-hour intervals (or according to agency policy). Notify physician for the following: sedation rating of 3, decrease in respiratory depth, and respiratory rate below 8 breaths/min.	
____	____	____	7. Keep head of bed elevated 30 degrees unless this is contraindicated.	
____	____	____	8. Record level of pain and effectiveness of pain relief.	
____	____	____	9. Monitor urinary output and assess for bladder distention.	
____	____	____	10. Assess motor strength every 4 hours.	
____	____	____	11. Monitor for adverse effects (pruritus, nausea, and vomiting).	
____	____	____	12. Assess for signs of infection at the insertion site.	
____	____	____	13. Change the dressing over the catheter exit site every 24 to 48 hours or as needed per agency policy. Change the infusion tubing every 48 hours or as specified by agency policy.	

Excellent	Satisfactory	Needs Practice	SKILL 10-4 **Caring for a Patient Receiving** **Epidural Analgesia** *(Continued)*	
				Comments
——	——	——	14. After providing care, remove and dispose of gloves and perform hand hygiene.	
——	——	——	15. Document catheter patency, condition of insertion site and dressing, vital signs and assessment information, and any change in infusion rate, solution, or tubing, analgesics administered, and patient's response.	

Skill Checklists to Accompany Taylor's Clinical Nursing Skills:
A Nursing Process Approach

Name _____   Date _____

Unit _____   Position _____

Instructor/Evaluator: _____   Position _____

SKILL 11-1
Inserting a Nasogastric Tube

Excellent	Satisfactory	Needs Practice	**Goal:** To pass a tube into the gastrointestinal tract for administration of a formula containing adequate nutrients without experiencing any complications.	Comments
____	____	____	1. Check physician's order for insertion of nasogastric tube.	
____	____	____	2. Explain procedure to patient, discussing with patient the need for the nasogastric tube; answer any questions patient may have.	
____	____	____	3. Gather equipment.	
____	____	____	4. If nasogastric tube is rubber, place it in a basin with ice for 5 to 10 minutes or place a plastic tube in a basin of warm water if needed.	
____	____	____	5. Perform hand hygiene. Don disposable gloves.	
____	____	____	6. Assist patient to high Fowler's position, or to 45 degrees if unable to maintain upright position, and drape chest with bath towel or disposable pad. Have emesis basin and tissues handy.	
____	____	____	7. Measure distance to insert the tube by placing tip of tube at patient's nostril and extending to tip of earlobe and then to tip of xiphoid process. Mark tube with a piece of tape.	
____	____	____	8. Lubricate tip of tube (at least 1 to 2 inches) with water-soluble lubricant. Apply topical analgesic to nostril and oropharynx or ask patient to hold ice chips in his or her mouth for several minutes.	
____	____	____	9. After having the patient lift his or her head, insert tube into nostril while directing tube upward and backward. Patient may gag when tube reaches the pharynx. Provide tissues for tearing or watering eyes.	
____	____	____	10. Instruct patient to touch his or her chin to chest. Encourage him or her to sip water through a straw or to swallow even if no fluids are permitted. Advance tube in a downward-and-backward direction when patient swallows. Stop when patient breathes. If gagging and coughing persist, check placement of tube with a tongue blade and flashlight. Keep advancing tube until tape marking is reached. Do not use force. Rotate tube if it meets resistance.	

Excellent	Satisfactory	Needs Practice		Comments
____	____	____	11. Discontinue the procedure and remove the tube if there are signs of distress, such as gasping, coughing, cyanosis, and the inability to speak or hum.	
____	____	____	12. While keeping one hand on tube, determine that the tube is in the patient's stomach.	
____	____	____	a. Attach syringe to end of tube and aspirate a small amount of stomach contents.	
____	____	____	b. Measure pH of paper or a meter.	
____	____	____	c. Visualize aspirated contents checking for color and consistency.	
____	____	____	d. Obtain radiograph of placement of tube (as ordered by physician).	
____	____	____	13. Apply tincture of benzoin to tip of nose and allow to dry. Secure tube with tape to patient's nose. Be careful not to pull tube too tightly against nose.	
____	____	____	a. Cut a 4-inch piece of tape and split bottom 2 inches, or use packaged nose tape for nasogastric tubes.	
____	____	____	b. Place unsplit end over bridge of patient's nose.	
____	____	____	c. Wrap split ends under tubing and up and over onto nose.	
____	____	____	14. Attach tube to suction or clamp tube and cap it according to physician's orders.	
____	____	____	15. Secure tube to patient's gown by using a rubber band or tape and a safety pin. If double-lumen tube is used, secure vent above stomach level. Attach at shoulder level.	
____	____	____	16. Assist or provide patient with oral hygiene at regular intervals.	
____	____	____	17. Remove disposable gloves and perform hand hygiene. Remove all equipment and make patient comfortable.	
____	____	____	18. Record the insertion procedure, type and size of tube, and measure tube from tip of nose to end of tube. Also document description of gastric contents, which naris used, and patient's response.	

Name _____   Date _____

Unit _____   Position _____

Instructor/Evaluator: _____   Position _____

Excellent	Satisfactory	Needs Practice	SKILL 11-2 **Administering a Tube Feeding** **Goal:** To provide enteral nutrition by administering formula at the prescribed rate or interval without causing patient nausea or vomiting.	Comments
___	___	___	1. Explain procedure to patient. Use a stethoscope to assess bowel sounds.	
___	___	___	2. Assemble equipment. Check amount, concentration, type, and frequency of tube feeding on patient's chart. Check expiration date of formula.	
___	___	___	3. Perform hand hygiene. Don disposable gloves.	
___	___	___	4. Position patient with head of bed elevated at least 30 degrees or as near normal position for eating as possible.	
___	___	___	5. Unpin tube from patient's gown and check to see that nasogastric tube is properly located in stomach, as described in Skill 11-1, Action 12.	
___	___	___	6. Aspirate all gastric contents with syringe and measure. Return immediately through tube, saving small amount to measure gastric pH. Flush tube with 30 mL of sterile water for irrigation. Proceed with feeding if amount of residual does not exceed policy of agency or physician's guideline. Disconnect syringe from tubing.	
			7. When using a feeding bag (open system):	
___	___	___	a. Hang bag on intravenous pole and adjust to about 12 inches above stomach. Clamp tubing.	
___	___	___	b. Cleanse top of feeding container with alcohol before opening it. Pour formula into feeding bag and allow solution to run through tubing. Close clamp.	
___	___	___	c. Attach feeding setup to feeding tube, open clamp, and regulate drip rate according to physician's order or allow feeding to run in over 30 minutes.	
___	___	___	d. Add 30 to 60 mL (1 to 2 ounces) of sterile water for irrigation to feeding bag when feeding is almost completed and allow it to run through tube.	
___	___	___	e. Clamp tubing immediately after water has been instilled. Disconnect from feeding tube. Clamp tube and cover end with sterile gauze secured with rubber band or apply cap.	

			SKILL 11-2	
Excellent	Satisfactory	Needs Practice	**Administering a Tube Feeding** *(Continued)*	**Comments**

Excellent	Satisfactory	Needs Practice		Comments
___	___	___	8. When using a large syringe (open system):	
___	___	___	a. Remove plunger from 30- or 60-mL syringe	
___	___	___	b. Attach syringe to feeding tube, pour premeasured amount of tube feeding into syringe, open clamp, and allow feeding to enter tube. Regulate the rate by raising or lowering the height of the syringe. Do not push formula with syringe plunger.	
___	___	___	c. Add 30 to 60 mL of water for irrigation to syringe when feeding is almost completed and allow it to run through the tube.	
___	___	___	d. When syringe has emptied, hold the syringe high and disconnect from the tube. Clamp the tube and cover end with a sterile gauze secured with a rubber band or apply a cap.	
___	___	___	9. When using prefilled tube feeding setup (closed system):	
___	___	___	a. Remove screw-on cap and attach administration setup with drip chamber and tubing. Hang set on intravenous pole and adjust to about 12 inches above the stomach. Clamp tubing and squeeze drip chamber to fill to one-third to one-half of capacity. Release clamp and run formula through tubing. Close clamp.	
___	___	___	b. Follow Actions 7c, 7d, and 7e. Feeding pump may be used with tube feeding setup to regulate drip.	
			For Continuous Feedings	
___	___	___	10. When using a feeding pump (continuous feeding):	
___	___	___	a. Close flow regulator clamp on tubing and fill feeding bag with prescribed formula. Amount depends on agency policy. Place label on container.	
___	___	___	b. Hang feeding container on intravenous pole and allow solution to flow through tubing.	
___	___	___	c. Connect to feeding pump following manufacturer's directions. Set rate.	
___	___	___	d. Check residual every 4 to 8 hours.	
___	___	___	11. Observe patient's response during and after tube feeding.	
___	___	___	12. Have patient remain in upright position for at least 30 to 60 minutes after feeding.	
___	___	___	13. Wash and clean equipment or replace according to agency policy. Remove gloves and perform hand hygiene.	
___	___	___	14. Record type and amount of feeding, residual amount, verification of placement, and patient's response. Monitor blood glucose, if ordered by physician.	

166

Skill Checklists to Accompany Taylor's Clinical Nursing Skills:
A Nursing Process Approach

Name _____ Date _____

Unit _____ Position _____

Instructor/Evaluator: _____ Position _____

Excellent	Satisfactory	Needs Practice	SKILL 11-3 **Removing a Nasogastric Tube**	Comments
			Goal: To promote comfort and prevent trauma to gastrointestinal tract.	
___	___	___	1. Check physician's order for removal of nasogastric tube.	
___	___	___	2. Explain procedure to patient and assist to semi-Fowler's position.	
___	___	___	3. Gather equipment.	
___	___	___	4. Perform hand hygiene. Don clean disposable gloves.	
___	___	___	5. Place towel or disposable pad across patient's chest. Give tissues and emesis basin to patient.	
___	___	___	6. Discontinue suction and separate tube from suction. Unpin tube from patient's gown and carefully remove adhesive tape from patient's nose.	
___	___	___	7. Attach syringe and flush with 10 mL water or normal saline solution or clear with 30 to 50 cc of air (optional).	
___	___	___	8. Instruct patient to take a deep breath and hold it.	
___	___	___	9. Clamp tube with fingers by doubling tube on itself. Quickly and carefully remove tube while patient holds breath.	
___	___	___	10. Dispose of tube per agency policy. Remove gloves and place in bag.	
___	___	___	11. Offer mouth care to patient and facial tissues to blow nose.	
___	___	___	12. Measure nasogastric drainage in suction device. Remove all equipment and dispose according to agency policy. Perform hand hygiene.	
___	___	___	13. Record removal of tube, patient's response, and measure of drainage. Continue to monitor patient for 2 to 4 hours after tube removal for gastric distention, nausea, or vomiting.	

Skill Checklists to Accompany Taylor's Clinical Nursing Skills:
A Nursing Process Approach

Name _____   Date _____

Unit _____   Position _____

Instructor/Evaluator: _____   Position _____

SKILL 11-4

Irrigating a Nasogastric Tube Connected to Suction

Goal: To maintain patency of gastrointestinal tube.

Excellent	Satisfactory	Needs Practice		Comments
___	___	___	1. Check physician's order for irrigation. Explain procedure to patient.	
___	___	___	2. Gather necessary equipment. Check expiration dates on irrigating solution and irrigation set.	
___	___	___	3. Perform hand hygiene. Don gloves.	
___	___	___	4. Assist patient to semi-Fowler's position, unless this is contraindicated.	
___	___	___	5. Check placement of nasogastric tube (see Skill 11-1, Action 12).	
___	___	___	6. Pour irrigating solution into container. Draw up 30 mL of saline solution (or amount ordered by physician) into syringe.	
___	___	___	7. Clamp suction tubing near connection site. Disconnect tube from suction apparatus and lay on disposable pad or towel or hold both tubes upright in nondominant hand.	
___	___	___	8. Place tip of syringe in tube. If Salem sump or double-lumen tube is used, make sure that syringe tip is placed in drainage port and not in blue air vent. Hold syringe upright and gently insert the irrigant (or allow solution to flow in by gravity, if agency or physician indicates). Do not force solution into tube.	
___	___	___	9. If unable to irrigate tube, reposition patient and attempt irrigation again. Check with physician if repeated attempts to irrigate tube fail.	
___	___	___	10. Withdraw or aspirate fluid into syringe. If no return, inject 20 cc of air and aspirate again.	
___	___	___	11. Reconnect tube to suction. Observe movement of solution or drainage. Remove gloves.	
___	___	___	12. Measure and record amount and description of irrigant and returned solution.	
___	___	___	13. Rinse equipment if it will be reused.	
___	___	___	14. Remove gloves; perform hand hygiene.	
___	___	___	15. Record irrigation procedure, description of drainage, and patient's response.	

Skill Checklists to Accompany Taylor's Clinical Nursing Skills:
A Nursing Process Approach

Name _____   Date _____

Unit _____   Position _____

Instructor/Evaluator: _____   Position _____

Excellent	Satisfactory	Needs Practice	SKILL 11-5 **Administering Medications via a Nasogastric Tube**	
			Goal: To administer medication via the tube with patient experiencing intended effect and remaining free of injury.	**Comments**
___	___	___	1. Check to see whether medications to be administered come in a liquid form. If pills or capsules are to be given, check with pharmacy about crushing or opening capsules. Ensure that the tube is patent and irrigate as necessary (see Skill 11-4).	
___	___	___	2. Using oral syringes, draw up all medications to be given. Also draw up a syringe containing 15 to 20 mL of water for each medication that is to be given.	
___	___	___	3. Perform hand hygiene and don gloves. If patient has continuous tube feedings, pause tube feeding pump.	
___	___	___	4. Fold tube over and clamp with fingers. Disconnect tubing for feeding from NG tube. Insert tip of 60-mL syringe into gastric tube. Release NG tube. Pull plunger back using a constant gentle pressure to check for residue.	
___	___	___	5. After noting amount, replace residual feeding back into stomach.	
___	___	___	6. Fold NG tube over and clamp with fingers. Remove 60-mL syringe. Apply syringe with first medication to be given.	
___	___	___	7. Release gastric tube and administer the medication. Clamp the gastric tube with fingers and remove syringe. Insert the syringe containing water into the tube and flush the tube with a constant delivery rate.	
___	___	___	8. Fold tubing back over and clamp with fingers. If more medications are to be given, repeat Actions 6 and 7. If no more medications are to be given, reconnect tube feeding. When last medication is administered, flush tube with 30 mL of water (or according to institution's policy). Unclamp gastric tube, and restart tube feeding.	
___	___	___	9. Remove gloves and perform hand hygiene.	
___	___	___	10. Record amount of water used to flush tube and document on the medication administration record.	

Skill Checklists to Accompany Taylor's Clinical Nursing Skills:
A Nursing Process Approach

Name _____   Date _____

Unit _____   Position _____

Instructor/Evaluator: _____   Position _____

Excellent	Satisfactory	Needs Practice	SKILL 11-6 **Caring for a Gastrostomy Tube**	
			Goal: To ensure patient ingests an adequate diet with no signs of irritation, excoriation, or infection at the tube insertion site.	**Comments**
____	____	____	1. Explain procedure to patient.	
____	____	____	2. Perform hand hygiene. Don disposable gloves.	
____	____	____	3. a. If the gastrostomy tube is new and still has sutures holding it in place: Dip cotton tipped applicator into sterile solution and gently cleanse around the insertion site removing any crust or drainage.	
____	____	____	b. If the gastric tube insertion site has healed and the sutures are removed: Wet a washcloth and apply a small amount of soap onto washcloth. Gently cleanse around the insertion removing any crust or drainage. Rinse site removing all soap.	
____	____	____	4. Pat skin around insertion site dry.	
____	____	____	5. If the sutures have been removed, rotate the guard or external bumper 90 degrees at least once a day.	
____	____	____	6. Remove gloves and perform hand hygiene.	
____	____	____	7. Record care given, including appearance of site, any drainage present, and patient's response.	

Skill Checklists to Accompany Taylor's Clinical Nursing Skills:
A Nursing Process Approach

Name _____ Date _____

Unit _____ Position _____

Instructor/Evaluator: _____ Position _____

Excellent	Satisfactory	Needs Practice	SKILL 11-7 **Monitoring the Blood Glucose Level**	Comments
			Goal: To keep patient blood glucose level within acceptable parameters while remaining free of injury.	
___	___	___	1. Check physician's order for monitoring schedule.	
___	___	___	2. Gather equipment.	
___	___	___	3. Explain procedure to patient and instruct the patient about the need for monitoring blood glucose.	
___	___	___	4. Perform hand hygiene. Don disposable gloves.	
___	___	___	5. Prepare lancet.	
___	___	___	6. Remove test strip from the vial and recap container immediately. Turn monitor and check that code number on strip matches the code number on the monitor screen.	
___	___	___	7. Massage side of finger for adult toward puncture site.	
___	___	___	8. Have patient wash hands with soap and warm water or cleanse area with alcohol. Dry thoroughly.	
___	___	___	9. Hold lancet perpendicular to skin and prick site with the lancet.	
___	___	___	10. Wipe away first drop of blood with cotton ball if recommended by manufacturer of monitor.	
___	___	___	11. Lightly squeeze or milk the puncture site until a hanging drop of blood has formed (check instructions for monitor).	
___	___	___	12. Gently touch drop of blood to pad on test strip without smearing it.	
___	___	___	13. Insert strip into the meter according to directions for that specific device. Some devices require that the drop of blood is applied to a test strip that has already been inserted in the monitor.	
___	___	___	14. Press time if directed by manufacturer.	
___	___	___	15. Apply pressure to puncture site with a cotton ball. Do not use alcohol wipe.	
___	___	___	16. Read blood glucose results and document appropriately at bedside. Inform patient of test result.	
___	___	___	17. Turn meter off, dispose of supplies appropriately, and place lancet in sharps container.	
___	___	___	18. Remove gloves and perform hand hygiene.	
___	___	___	19. Record blood glucose on chart or medication record. Report abnormal results to physician.	

Skill Checklists to Accompany Taylor's Clinical Nursing Skills:
A Nursing Process Approach

Name _____   Date _____

Unit _____   Position _____

Instructor/Evaluator: _____   Position _____

SKILL 12-1

Offering and Removing a Bedpan or Urinal

Goal: To provide privacy while assisting a bedridden patient to void or defecate.

Excellent	Satisfactory	Needs Practice		Comments
___	___	___	1. Bring bedpan or urinal and equipment to bedside. Perform hand hygiene and don disposable gloves.	
___	___	___	2. Warm bedpan, if it is made of metal, by rinsing with warm water.	
___	___	___	3. Place adjustable bed in the high position.	
___	___	___	4. Place bedpan or urinal on chair next to bed or on foot of bed. Fold top linen back just enough to allow placement of bedpan or urinal. If there is no waterproof pad on the bedpan and time allows, consider placing a waterproof pad under patient's buttocks before placing bedpan or urinal.	
___	___	___	5. If patient needs assistance to move onto bedpan, have him or her bend knees and rest some of his or her weight on heels. Assist patient by placing one hand under lower back and slip bedpan into place with the other hand.	
___	___	___	6. If patient is unable to lift, the patient may be placed on his or her side, bedpan placed against buttocks, and patient rolled back onto bedpan.	
___	___	___	7. Ensure that bedpan is in its proper position, with patient's buttocks resting on the rounded shelf of bedpan. For male patients, urinal is properly placed between slightly spread legs with penis positioned in it and with urinal resting on bed. If patient has voided more than 500 mL in the past, urinal opening should be slightly raised.	
___	___	___	8. If permitted, raise head of the bed as near to the sitting position as tolerated. Cover with bed linens.	
___	___	___	9. Place call device and toilet tissue within easy reach. Leave patient if it is safe to do so. Use side rails appropriately. Remove gloves and perform hand hygiene.	
___	___	___	10. Perform hand hygiene and don disposable gloves. Remove bedpan in the same manner in which it was offered, being careful to hold it steady. If necessary to assist patient, wrap tissue around the hand several times and wipe patient clean, using one stroke from the pubic area	

Excellent	Satisfactory	Needs Practice	SKILL 12-1 **Offering and Removing a Bedpan or Urinal** *(Continued)*	Comments
			toward the anal area. Discard tissue and use more until patient is clean. Place the patient on his or her side and spread buttocks to clean anal area. Cover bedpan.	
___	___	___	11. Do not place toilet tissue in bedpan if a specimen is required or if measurement of elimination is required. Have receptacle handy for discarding tissue.	
___	___	___	12. Offer patient supplies to wash and dry his or her hands, assisting as necessary.	
___	___	___	13. Empty and clean bedpan and urinal. Perform hand hygiene. Record according to agency procedure. Recording may be done on Intake/Output record.	

Skill Checklists to Accompany Taylor's Clinical Nursing Skills:
A Nursing Process Approach

Name _____ Date _____

Unit _____ Position _____

Instructor/Evaluator: _____ Position _____

Excellent	Satisfactory	Needs Practice	SKILL 12-2 **Catheterizing the Female Urinary Bladder** **(Straight and Indwelling)** **Goal:** To safely introduce catheter into bladder to promote urine drainage.	Comments
___	___	___	1. Assemble equipment. Perform hand hygiene. Explain procedure and purpose to patient. Discuss any allergies with patient, especially iodine or latex.	
___	___	___	2. Provide good light. Artificial light is recommended (use of flashlight requires an assistant to hold and position it).	
___	___	___	3. Provide privacy by closing curtains or door.	
___	___	___	4. Assist patient to the dorsal recumbent position with knees flexed and feet about 2 feet apart. Drape patient. Or, if preferable, place patient in the side-lying position. Slide waterproof drape under patient.	
___	___	___	5. Don disposable gloves. Spread the labia well with fingers and clean the area at the vaginal orifice with a washcloth and warm water, using a different corner of the washcloth with each stroke. Wipe from above the orifice downward toward sacrum (front to back). Rinse and dry. Perform hand hygiene again.	
___	___	___	6. Prepare urine drainage setup if indwelling catheter is to be inserted and if a separate urine collection system is used. Secure to bed frame according to manufacturer's directions.	
___	___	___	7. Open sterile catheterization tray on a clean overbed table using sterile technique.	
___	___	___	8. Put on sterile gloves. Grasp upper corners of drape and unfold without touching unsterile areas. Fold back a corner on each side to make a cuff over gloved hands. Ask patient to lift her buttocks. Slide sterile drape under her with gloves protected by cuff.	
___	___	___	9. A fenestrated sterile drape may be placed over perineal area, exposing the labia.	
___	___	___	10. Place sterile tray on drape between patient's thighs.	
___	___	___	11. Open all supplies.	
___	___	___	a. If catheter is to be indwelling, test catheter balloon. Remove protective cap on tip of syringe and attach syringe prefilled with sterile water to injection port.	

Excellent	Satisfactory	Needs Practice	SKILL 12-2 **Catheterizing the Female Urinary Bladder** **(Straight and Indwelling)** *(Continued)*	
				Comments
			Inject appropriate amount of fluid. If balloon inflates properly, withdraw fluid and leave syringe attached to port.	
___	___	___	b. Fluff cotton balls in tray before pouring antiseptic solution over them. Open specimen container if specimen is to be obtained.	
___	___	___	c. Lubricate 1 to 2 inches of catheter tip.	
___	___	___	12. With thumb and one finger of your nondominant hand, spread labia and identify meatus. Be prepared to maintain separation of labia with one hand until catheter is inserted and urine is flowing well and continuously.	
___	___	___	13. Using cotton balls held with forceps, move cotton ball from above the meatus down toward the rectum. Clean both labial folds and then directly over the meatus. Discard each cotton ball after one downward stroke.	
___	___	___	14. With uncontaminated gloved hand, place drainage end of the catheter in receptacle. For insertion of an indwelling catheter that is preattached to sterile tubing and drainage container (closed drainage system), position catheter and setup within easy reach on the sterile field. Ensure clamp on drainage bag is closed.	
___	___	___	15. Insert catheter tip into the meatus 5 to 7.5 cm (2 to 3 inches) or until urine flows. Do not use force to push catheter through the urethra into the bladder. Ask patient to breathe deeply. Rotate catheter gently if slight resistance is met as catheter reaches the external sphincter. For an indwelling catheter: Once urine drains, advance catheter another 2.5 to 5.0 cm (1 to 2 inches).	
___	___	___	16. Hold catheter securely with the nondominant hand while bladder empties. Collect specimen if required. Specimen should be caught in middle of flow. After 50 to 100 mL of urine have drained, place specimen collection device under the opening of the catheter and allow urine to drain into container. When enough urine has been caught, remove specimen container. Continue drainage according to agency policy.	
___	___	___	17. Remove catheter smoothly and slowly if a straight catheterization was ordered.	
___	___	___	18. If the catheter is to be indwelling:	
___	___	___	a. Inflate balloon according to manufacturer's recommendations. Inject the entire volume supplied in the prefilled syringe.	

SKILL 12-2
Catheterizing the Female Urinary Bladder
(Straight and Indwelling) *(Continued)*

Excellent	Satisfactory	Needs Practice		Comments
——	——	——	b. Tug gently on catheter after balloon is inflated to feel resistance.	
——	——	——	c. Attach catheter to drainage system if necessary.	
——	——	——	d. Secure to upper thigh with a Velcro leg strap or tape. Leave some slack in catheter to allow for leg movement.	
——	——	——	e. Check that drainage tubing is not kinked and that movement of side rails does not interfere with catheter or drainage bag.	
——	——	——	19. Remove equipment and make patient comfortable in bed. Care for equipment according to agency policy. Send urine specimen to laboratory promptly or refrigerate it.	
——	——	——	20. Perform perineal care as described in Action 5.	
——	——	——	21. Remove gloves from inside out. Perform hand hygiene.	
——	——	——	22. Record time of catheterization, state of catheter and balloon, amount of urine removed, description of urine, if a specimen was sent, and patient's reaction to procedure in the medical record; also document the urine amount on the intake and output flow sheet.	

Name _____   Date _____

Unit _____   Position _____

Instructor/Evaluator: _____   Position _____

Excellent	Satisfactory	Needs Practice	SKILL 12-3 **Catheterizing the Male Urinary Bladder** **(Straight and Indwelling)**	
			Goal: To safely introduce catheter into bladder to promote urine drainage.	**Comments**
___	___	___	1. Follow Actions 1 to 3 for female catheterization in Skill 12-2.	
___	___	___	2. Position patient on his back with thighs slightly apart. Drape patient so that only area around penis is exposed.	
___	___	___	3. Clean the penile area as in Action five. Follow Actions 5 through 7 for female catheterization in Skill 12-2.	
___	___	___	4. Put on sterile gloves. Open sterile drape and place on patient's thighs. Place the fenestrated drape with the opening over penis.	
___	___	___	5. Place catheter set on or next to patient's legs on the sterile drape.	
___	___	___	6. Open all supplies.	
___	___	___	a. If catheter is to be indwelling, test catheter balloon. Remove protective cap on tip of syringe and attach syringe prefilled with sterile water to the injection port. Inject appropriate amount of fluid. If balloon inflates properly, withdraw fluid and leave syringe attached to port.	
___	___	___	b. Fluff cotton balls before pouring antiseptic solution over cotton balls or gauze. Open specimen container if specimen is to be obtained.	
___	___	___	c. Remove cap from syringe prefilled with lubricant.	
___	___	___	7. Lift penis with your nondominant hand, which is then considered contaminated. Retract foreskin in the uncircumcised male patient. Clean area at meatus with cotton ball held with forceps. Use circular motion, moving from the meatus toward base of the penis for three cleansings.	
___	___	___	8. Hold the penis with slight upward tension and perpendicular to patient's body. Gently insert tip of syringe with lubricant into urethra and instill 10 mL of lubricant. If kit in use does not have prefilled syringe, lubricate catheter tip.	

Catheterizing the Male Urinary Bladder
(Straight and Indwelling) *(Continued)*

Excellent	Satisfactory	Needs Practice		Comments
——	——	——	9. With your dominant hand, place drainage end of catheter in the receptacle. For insertion of indwelling catheter that is preattached to sterile tubing and drainage container (closed drainage system), position the catheter and setup within easy reach on the sterile field. Check to make sure that clamp on drainage bag is closed.	
——	——	——	10. Ask patient to bear down as if voiding. Insert the tip into the meatus. Advance catheter 15 to 20 cm (6 to 8 inches) or until urine flows. Do not use force to introduce the catheter. If the catheter resists entry, ask patient to breathe deeply and rotate catheter slightly. For an indwelling catheter, once urine drains, advance catheter to the bifurcation of the catheter. Once balloon is inflated, catheter may be gently pulled back into place. Replace the foreskin over catheter. Lower the penis.	
——	——	——	11. Follow Actions 16 through 20 for female catheterization in Skill 12-2 except that the catheter may be secured to the upper thigh or lower abdomen with the penis directed toward the patient's chest. Slack should be left in the catheter to prevent tension.	
——	——	——	12. Remove gloves from inside out. Perform hand hygiene.	
——	——	——	13. Record the time of the catheterization, catheter and balloon size, the amount of urine removed, a description of the urine, if a specimen was sent, and the patient's reaction to the procedure in the medical record; also document the urine amount on the intake and output flow sheet.	

Skill Checklists to Accompany Taylor's Clinical Nursing Skills:
A Nursing Process Approach

Name _____   Date _____

Unit _____   Position _____

Instructor/Evaluator: _____   Position _____

Excellent	Satisfactory	Needs Practice	SKILL 12-4 **Irrigating the Catheter Using the Closed System**	Comments
			Goal: To restore or maintain patency of an indwelling catheter through intermittent flushing of the tube.	
___	___	___	1. Assemble equipment. Perform hand hygiene. Explain the procedure and its purpose to patient.	
___	___	___	2. Provide privacy by closing curtains or door and draping patient with bath blanket.	
___	___	___	3. Assist patient to a comfortable position and expose the aspiration port on the catheter setup. Place a waterproof drape under catheter and aspiration port.	
___	___	___	4. Open the sterile supplies. Pour sterile solution into sterile basin. Aspirate irrigant (30 to 50 mL) into the sterile syringe and attach capped sterile needle. Don gloves.	
___	___	___	5. Wipe the aspiration port with alcohol swabs or gauze square with antiseptic solution.	
___	___	___	6. Clamp or fold catheter tubing distal to aspiration port.	
___	___	___	7. Remove cap and insert needle into port. Gently instill solution into catheter.	
___	___	___	8. Remove needle from port. Unclamp or unfold tubing and allow irrigant and urine to drain. Repeat procedure as necessary.	
___	___	___	9. Remove equipment and discard uncapped needle and syringe in appropriate receptacle. Remove gloves and perform hand hygiene. Make patient comfortable.	
___	___	___	10. Assess the patient's response to the procedure and the quality and amount of drainage with the irrigation. Document on patient's chart.	
___	___	___	11. Record amount of irrigant used on Intake/Output record. Subtract this from urine output when totaled.	

Skill Checklists to Accompany Taylor's Clinical Nursing Skills:
A Nursing Process Approach

Name _____   Date _____

Unit _____   Position _____

Instructor/Evaluator: _____   Position _____

			SKILL 12-5	
Excellent	**Satisfactory**	**Needs Practice**	**Giving a Continuous Bladder Irrigation** **Goal:** To restore or maintain patency of indwelling catheter through continuous flushing of tube.	**Comments**
___	___	___	1. Explain procedure and purpose to patient.	
___	___	___	2. Assemble equipment and double-check physician's order.	
___	___	___	3. Perform hand hygiene.	
___	___	___	4. Provide privacy by closing curtains or door and draping patient with bath blanket.	
___	___	___	5. Prepare the sterile irrigation bag for use as directed by manufacturer. Secure clamp and attach sterile tubing with drip chamber to container. Hang bag on intravenous pole 2.5 to 3 feet above level of patient's bladder. Release clamp and remove protective cover on end of tubing without contaminating it. Allow solution to flush tubing and remove air. Reclamp.	
___	___	___	6. Don gloves. Using sterile technique, attach irrigation tubing to the irrigation port of the three-way Foley catheter. If a closed system is used, tubing may already be connected to irrigation port on the catheter.	
___	___	___	7. Release the clamp on the irrigation tubing and regulate flow according to physician's order. At times, physician may order bladder irrigation to be done with a medicated solution. In these cases, using an intravenous pump to regulate flow is recommended.	
___	___	___	8. As irrigation is completed, clamp tubing. Do not allow drip chamber to empty. Disconnect empty bag and attach full irrigation bag. Continue as ordered by physician.	
___	___	___	9. Assess patient's response to procedure and the quality and amount of drainage. Document on patient's chart.	
___	___	___	10. Record amount of irrigant used on Intake/Output record. Don gloves and empty drainage collection bag as each new container is hung and recorded.	
___	___	___	11. Remove gloves and perform hand hygiene.	

Skill Checklists to Accompany Taylor's Clinical Nursing Skills:
A Nursing Process Approach

Name _____   Date _____

Unit _____   Position _____

Instructor/Evaluator: _____   Position _____

SKILL 12-6
Applying a Condom Catheter

Goal: To safely apply an external device to penis to collect urine.

Excellent	Satisfactory	Needs Practice		Comments
___	___	___	1. Explain procedure to patient. Obtain a latex-free condom if patient is allergic to latex.	
___	___	___	2. Prepare urinary drainage setup or reusable leg bag for attachment to condom sheath.	
___	___	___	3. Perform hand hygiene.	
___	___	___	4. Assist patient to the supine position. Close the curtain or door. Use a bath blanket and sheet to expose only patient's genital area.	
___	___	___	5. Don disposable gloves. Trim any long pubic hair that is in contact with the penis.	
___	___	___	6. Wash genital area with soap and water, rinse, and dry thoroughly. If uncircumcised, retract foreskin and clean the glans of the penis. Replace foreskin.	
___	___	___	7. Roll the condom sheath outward onto itself. Grasp the penis firmly with your nondominant hand. Apply condom sheath by rolling it onto penis with your dominant hand. Leave a 2.5- to 5-cm (1- to 2-inch) space between the tip of the penis and the end of the condom sheath.	
___	___	___	8. Apply the elastic or Velcro strap in a snug but not too tight manner. Do not allow elastic or Velcro to come in contact with skin.	
___	___	___	9. Connect the condom sheath to the drainage setup. Avoid kinking or twisting drainage tubing.	
___	___	___	10. Remove equipment. Place patient in a comfortable safe position. Perform hand hygiene.	
___	___	___	11. Assess the patient's response and record observations on the patient's record.	

Skill Checklists to Accompany Taylor's Clinical Nursing Skills:
A Nursing Process Approach

Name _____   Date _____

Unit _____   Position _____

Instructor/Evaluator: _____   Position _____

Excellent	Satisfactory	Needs Practice	SKILL 12-7 **Changing a Stoma Appliance on an Ileal Conduit** **Goal:** To facilitate urine collection and stoma assessment of a surgically created urinary diversion.	Comments
____	____	____	1. Explain procedure and encourage patient to observe or participate if possible. Have patient perform hand hygiene. Provide for privacy.	
____	____	____	2. Assemble equipment.	
____	____	____	3. Perform hand hygiene and don disposable gloves.	
____	____	____	4. Have patient sit or stand, if able, to assist with skill or assume supine position in bed.	
____	____	____	5. Empty pouch being worn into graduated container (before removing if it is reusable and not attached to straight drainage).	
____	____	____	6. Gently remove pouch faceplate from the skin by pushing skin from appliance rather than pulling appliance from skin.	
____	____	____	7. Discard pouch appropriately, if disposable, or wash reusable pouch in lukewarm soap and water and allow to air dry.	
____	____	____	8. Clean skin around stoma with soap and water or commercial cleaner using washcloth or cotton balls. Make sure you remove all old adhesive from skin. An adhesive remover may be used.	
____	____	____	9. Gently pat dry. Make sure skin around stoma is thoroughly dry. Assess stoma and condition of surrounding skin.	
____	____	____	10. Place a gauze square or two over stoma opening.	
____	____	____	11. Apply a skin protectant to a 5-cm (2-inch) radius around stoma and allow it to dry completely, which takes about 30 seconds.	
____	____	____	12. If necessary, enlarge the size of the faceplate opening to fit the stoma.	
____	____	____	13. Remove gauze squares from stoma before applying pouch. Apply adhesive to faceplate or remove protective covering from disposable faceplate. Carefully position	

Excellent	Satisfactory	Needs Practice	SKILL 12-7 **Changing a Stoma Appliance on an Ileal Conduit** *(Continued)*	
				Comments
			appliance and press in place, moving from the center outward.	
___	___	___	14. Secure optional belt to appliance and around patient.	
___	___	___	15. Remove or discard equipment and assess patient's response to the procedure. Remove gloves and perform hand hygiene.	
___	___	___	16. Record appearance of the stoma and surrounding skin as well as patient reaction to procedure.	

Skill Checklists to Accompany Taylor's Clinical Nursing Skills:
A Nursing Process Approach

Name _____ Date _____

Unit _____ Position _____

Instructor/Evaluator: _____ Position _____

Excellent	Satisfactory	Needs Practice	SKILL 12-8 **Collecting a Urine Specimen for Culture** **Goal:** To obtain an adequate amount of urine from patient without contamination.	Comments
___	___	___	1. Explain procedure to patient, including performance of hand hygiene before and after specimen collection. Instruct patient to wipe perineal area from front to back or meatus of penis with moist towelette. Instruct a male patient who is not circumcised to retract the foreskin and clean the glans of the penis.	
___	___	___	2. Have patient void around 25 mL into toilet, stop stream, collect specimen (10 to 20 mL is more than enough), and then finish voiding. Tell patient not to touch the inside of the container or the lid.	
___	___	___	3. Have patient place lid on container. Done gloves and label container with patient's name, date, time, and person collecting specimen.	
___	___	___	4. Place container in biohazard bag. Remove gloves and perform hand hygiene.	
___	___	___	5. Transport specimen to laboratory as soon as possible. If unable to take specimen to laboratory immediately, refrigerate the specimen.	
___	___	___	6. Document specimen sent, odor, amount (if known), color, and clarity of urine.	
			For Very Young Children and Infants	
___	___	___	7. Explain steps to a young child, if old enough, and to the parent(s). Talk to the child at the child's level, stressing to the child and parents that there is no pain involved.	
___	___	___	8. Perform hand hygiene and don disposable gloves.	
___	___	___	9. Remove an infant's diaper. Perform thorough perineal care: for girls spread the labia and cleanse area and for boys retract foreskin if intact and cleanse glans of penis. Pat skin dry. For a young child, if old enough, follow the steps as for an adult.	
___	___	___	10. Remove paper backing from adhesive faceplate. Apply faceplate over labia or over penis. Gently push faceplate so that seal forms on infant's or younger child's skin. The	

			SKILL 12-8

Collecting a Urine Specimen for Culture *(Continued)*

Excellent	Satisfactory	Needs Practice		Comments
			inside of the bag is considered sterile. Take care to not contaminate the inside of the bag when applying.	
___	___	___	11. Apply clean diaper over bag. Remove gloves and perform hand hygiene. Check bag frequently to see if child has voided.	
___	___	___	12. As soon as enough urine is obtained in collection bag, perform hand hygiene and don gloves. Gently remove bag by pushing skin away from bag. Using sterile scissors, cut corner of bag and pour urine into sterile container.	
___	___	___	13. Perform perineal care for child and reapply diaper.	
___	___	___	14. Follow Actions 3 through 6 in the adult section of the procedure.	
			For the Patient with an Indwelling Urinary Catheter	
___	___	___	15. Explain procedure to patient. Organize equipment at bedside.	
___	___	___	16. Perform hand hygiene and don disposable gloves.	
___	___	___	17. Clamp or kink off the drainage tubing near the urinary catheter. Remove lid from specimen container ensuring to keep the inside of the container and lid from contamination.	
___	___	___	18. Cleanse aspirator port with the alcohol wipe, allowing the port to air dry.	
___	___	___	19. Insert the blunt-tipped needle into the port. Slowly aspirate enough urine for specimen culture (usually 5 mL will be adequate). Remove blunt-tipped needle from port.	
___	___	___	20. Slowly inject the urine into the specimen container. Replace the lid on the container. Dispose of the needle and syringe appropriately.	
___	___	___	21. Perform Actions 3 through 6 in the adult section of this procedure.	

Skill Checklists to Accompany Taylor's Clinical Nursing Skills:
A Nursing Process Approach

Name _____   Date _____

Unit _____   Position _____

Instructor/Evaluator: _____   Position _____

Excellent	Satisfactory	Needs Practice	SKILL 12-9 **Caring for a Suprapubic Catheter** **Goal:** To enable patient to eliminate adequate amounts of urine and keep skin around catheter free of redness, irritation, and excoriation.	Comments
——	——	——	1. Explain the procedure and encourage the patient to observe or participate if possible. Provide for privacy.	
——	——	——	2. Assemble the equipment.	
——	——	——	3. Perform hand hygiene and don disposable gloves.	
——	——	——	4. Wet washcloth and soap with warm water. Gently cleanse around the suprapubic exit site. Remove any encrustations present. If this is a new suprapubic catheter, use cotton-tipped applicators and sterile saline for cleaning until the incision has healed.	
——	——	——	5. Rinse area of all soap. Pat dry.	
——	——	——	6. If the exit site has been draining, place a small drain sponge around the catheter to absorb any drainage. Be prepared to change this sponge throughout the day depending on the amount of drainage. Do not cut a 4″ × 4″ gauze pad to make a drain sponge.	
——	——	——	7. Form a loop in the tubing and place tape on abdomen.	
——	——	——	8. Remove or discard the equipment and assess the patient's response to the procedure. Remove gloves and perform hand hygiene.	
——	——	——	9. Record the appearance of the catheter exit site and the surrounding skin, urine amount, and urine characteristics as well as the patient's reaction to the procedure.	

Skill Checklists to Accompany Taylor's Clinical Nursing Skills:
A Nursing Process Approach

Name _____   Date _____

Unit _____   Position _____

Instructor/Evaluator: _____   Position _____

SKILL 12-10

Caring for a Peritoneal Dialysis Catheter

Goal: To complete peritoneal dialysis catheter dressing change using aseptic technique without causing trauma to the site or patient.

Excellent	Satisfactory	Needs Practice		Comments
___	___	___	1. Explain procedure to patient. Close the curtain or door.	
___	___	___	2. Gather equipment. Perform hand hygiene and don nonsterile gloves.	
___	___	___	3. Assist the patient to the supine position. Expose the patient's abdomen.	
___	___	___	4. Don face mask; have patient put on face mask.	
___	___	___	5. Gently remove old dressing, noting for any odor, amount and color of drainage, leakage, and condition of skin around dialysis catheter.	
___	___	___	6. Remove nonsterile gloves. Set up sterile field. Open packages. Place two sterile 4″ × 4″ gauze pads in basin with hydrogen peroxide. Leave one sterile 4″ × 4″ gauze pad opened on sterile field. Don sterile gloves.	
___	___	___	7. Gently palpate the area surrounding the peritoneal dialysis catheter (PDC) exit site with the gauze soaked in hydrogen peroxide.	
___	___	___	8. Pick up PDC with nondominant hand. With the hydrogen peroxide–soaked gauze, cleanse the skin around the PDC exit site using a circular motion and starting at the PDC exit site and then slowly going outward 3 to 4 inches.	
___	___	___	9. Continue to hold PDC with nondominant hand. After the skin has dried, apply povidone-iodine to the catheter beginning at the PDC exit site, going around the catheter, and then moving up to the end of the catheter.	
___	___	___	10. Place drain sponge around the PDC exit site. Then place a 4″ × 4″ gauze pad over PDC exit site. Secure edges of gauze pad with tape. Some institutions recommend placing a transparent dressing over the gauze pads instead of tape.	
___	___	___	11. Remove sterile gloves and perform hand hygiene.	
___	___	___	12. Document the dressing change, including the condition of the skin surrounding the PDC exit site, drainage, or odor as well as the patient's reaction to the procedure.	

Skill Checklists to Accompany Taylor's Clinical Nursing Skills:
A Nursing Process Approach

Name _____   Date _____

Unit _____   Position _____

Instructor/Evaluator: _____   Position _____

SKILL 12-11

Caring for a Hemodialysis Access
(Arteriovenous Fistula or Graft)

Excellent	Satisfactory	Needs Practice	**Goal:** To maintain a patent graft or fistula.	Comments
——	——	——	1. Inspect area over access site for any redness, warmth, tenderness, or any skin blemishes. Palpate over access site feeling for a "thrill" or a vibration. Auscultate over access site listening for a "bruit" or a vibration.	
——	——	——	2. Ensure that sign is placed over head of bed informing other members of the health care team of which arm is affected. Do not perform a venipuncture or start an intravenous line on the access arm.	
——	——	——	3. Instruct the patient not to sleep with access arm under head or body.	
——	——	——	4. Instruct the patient not to lift heavy objects, carry heavy bags, including purses on the shoulder, on the access arm, or put pressure on the access arm.	
——	——	——	5. Document assessment findings and any patient education performed.	

Skill Checklists to Accompany Taylor's Clinical Nursing Skills:
A Nursing Process Approach

Name _____   Date _____

Unit _____   Position _____

Instructor/Evaluator: _____   Position _____

Excellent	Satisfactory	Needs Practice	SKILL 13-1 **Testing Stool for Occult Blood**	Comments
			Goal: To achieve a stool sample, with patient demonstrating ability to test stool (if indicated).	
___	___	___	1. Discuss with patient the need for a stool sample. Explain to patient the process in which the stool will be collected: either from a bowel movement or from a digital rectal examination. If specimen is from a bowel movement, instruct patient not to urinate or discard toilet paper with the stool, which may contaminate the specimen. Gather necessary equipment. • If stool sample is to be obtained from digital rectal examination, proceed to Action 2. • If stool sample is to be collected with a bowel movement, proceed to Action 9.	
___	___	___	2. If digital rectal examination is to be performed, perform hand hygiene and put on nonsterile gloves.	
___	___	___	3. If patient is able to stand, instruct patient to bend over examination table or bed placed at a comfortable height. If patient is bedridden, place in Sims or side-lying position.	
___	___	___	4. Generously lubricate 1 to 1½ inches of finger with water-soluble lubricant to be inserted into anus to collect stool sample.	
___	___	___	5. Ask patient to take a large deep breath through the nose and exhale through the mouth.	
___	___	___	6. After separating buttocks with nondominate hand, gently insert lubricated finger of dominate hand 1 to 2 inches into rectum while lightly palpating for any stool.	
___	___	___	7. Remove finger. Apply stool to one window of hemoccult testing card.	
___	___	___	8. Apply stool to second window of hemoccult testing card from different place on glove than first sample. *Skip to Actions 12 through 16.*	
___	___	___	9. If patient is to defecate for the stool sample, assist patient to bathroom, bedside commode, or place on bedpan. Instruct patient not to void or discard toilet paper into stool collection container.	

Testing Stool for Occult Blood *(Continued)*

Excellent	Satisfactory	Needs Practice		Comments
____	____	____	10. Perform hand hygiene and put on disposable gloves.	
____	____	____	11. With wooden applicator, apply a small amount of stool onto one window of the hemoccult testing card. With opposite end of wooden applicator, obtain another sample of stool from an alternate area and apply a small amount of stool onto second window of the hemoccult testing card.	
____	____	____	12. Close flap over stool samples.	
____	____	____	13. Open flap on opposite side of card and place two drops of developer over each window and wait the time as stated in the manufacturer's instructions.	
____	____	____	14. Observe card for any blue-colored areas.	
____	____	____	15. Discard hemoccult testing slide. Remove disposable gloves from inside out and discard. Perform hand hygiene.	
____	____	____	16. Document testing results.	

Skill Checklists to Accompany Taylor's Clinical Nursing Skills:
A Nursing Process Approach

Name _____   Date _____

Unit _____   Position _____

Instructor/Evaluator: _____   Position _____

Excellent	Satisfactory	Needs Practice	SKILL 13-2 **Inserting a Rectal Tube**	
			Goal: To decrease the level of pain experienced due to retained flatus.	**Comments**
___	___	___	1. Explain the technique for insertion of the rectal tube and the rationale for insertion to the patient. Gather the equipment.	
___	___	___	2. Perform hand hygiene and put on nonsterile gloves.	
___	___	___	3. Place patient in a side-lying position. Drape the patient properly to provide privacy and warmth.	
___	___	___	4. Lubricate approximately 4 inches (10 cm) of the rectal tube with water-soluble lubricant.	
___	___	___	5. Separate the buttocks so that anus is visible. Have patient take a slow deep breath, inhaling through nose and exhaling through mouth. Gently insert the rectal tube beyond the anal canal into the rectum approximately 4 inches (10 cm) for an adult. Use a shorter distance for a child depending on size.	
___	___	___	6. Secure a waterproof pad to the end of the rectal tube or place end of rectal tube into urinal.	
___	___	___	7. Leave the rectal tube in place for no longer than 20 minutes. Tube may be taped in place.	
___	___	___	8. Monitor patient for any change in heart rate while tube is in place.	
___	___	___	9. If patient is able, have them assume the prone or knee-chest position.	
___	___	___	10. Replace nonsterile gloves if they have been removed.	
___	___	___	11. Have patient take a slow deep breath, inhaling through nose and exhaling through mouth while removing rectal tube.	
___	___	___	12. Wrap contaminated end of rectal tube in paper towel and discard.	
___	___	___	13. Clean patient's perineal area.	
___	___	___	14. Remove disposable gloves from inside out and discard. Perform hand hygiene.	
___	___	___	15. Reassess abdomen: girth, percussion, and palpation.	

Inserting a Rectal Tube *(Continued)*

Excellent	Satisfactory	Needs Practice		Comments
___	___	___	16. Document the following: size of rectal tube used; length of time rectal tube left in place; color, amount, and consistency of any stool removed; any changes noted in abdominal girth, abdominal assessment or complaints of pain, patient's positions during procedure; and patient's reaction to procedure.	

Skill Checklists to Accompany Taylor's Clinical Nursing Skills:
A Nursing Process Approach

Name _____   Date _____

Unit _____   Position _____

Instructor/Evaluator: _____   Position _____

Excellent	Satisfactory	Needs Practice	SKILL 13-3 **Administering a Cleansing Enema**	Comments
			Goal: To introduce solution into large intestine to promote expulsion of feces.	
___	___	___	1. Verify physician's orders; gather the necessary equipment, and explain the enema procedure to the patient, including where he or she will defecate. Have bedpan, commode, or nearby bathroom ready for use.	
___	___	___	2. Warm solution in amount ordered, and check temperature with a bath thermometer if available. (If bath thermometer is not available, warm to room temperature or slightly higher and test on inner wrist.) If tap water is used, adjust temperature as it flows from faucet.	
___	___	___	3. Perform hand hygiene.	
___	___	___	4. Add enema solution to container. Release clamp and allow fluid to progress through tube before reclamping.	
___	___	___	5. Position waterproof pad under patient.	
___	___	___	6. Provide privacy. Position and drape patient on the left side (Sims position) with anus exposed or on back, as dictated by patient comfort and condition.	
___	___	___	7. Put on nonsterile gloves.	
___	___	___	8. Elevate solution so it is no higher than 45 cm (18 inches) above level of patient's anus. Plan to administer solution slowly over a period of 5 to 10 minutes. Container may be hung on an intravenous pole or held in nurse's hands at the proper height.	
___	___	___	9. Generously lubricate the last 5 to 7 cm (2 to 3 inches) of the rectal tube. A disposable enema set may have a prelubricated rectal tube.	
___	___	___	10. Lift buttock to expose anus. Slowly and gently insert enema tube 7 to 10 cm (3 to 4 inches). Direct it at an angle pointing toward the spine, not bladder. Ask patient to take several deep breaths.	
___	___	___	11. If tube meets resistance while inserting it, permit a small amount of solution to enter, withdraw tube slightly, and then continue to insert it. Do not force tube entry. Ask patient to take several deep breaths.	

KILL 13-3
Administering a Cleansing Enema *(Continued)*

Excellent	Satisfactory	Needs Practice		Comments
___	___	___	12. Introduce solution slowly over a period of 5 to 10 minutes. Hold tubing all the time solution is being instilled.	
___	___	___	13. Clamp tubing or lower container if patient has the desire to defecate or cramping occurs. Patient may also may be instructed to take small fast breaths or to pant.	
___	___	___	14. After solution has been given, clamp tubing and remove tube. Have paper towel ready to receive tube as it is withdrawn. Have patient retain solution until the urge to defecate becomes strong, usually in about 5 to 15 minutes.	
___	___	___	15. Remove nonsterile gloves from inside out and discard.	
___	___	___	16. When patient has a strong urge to defecate, place him or her in a sitting position on bedpan or assist to commode or bathroom. Stay with the patient or have call light readily accessible.	
___	___	___	17. Record character of the stool and patient's response to the enema. Remind patient not to flush commode before nurse inspects results of enema.	
___	___	___	18. Assist patient, if necessary, with cleaning of anal area. Offer washcloths, soap, and water to wash his or her hands.	
___	___	___	19. Leave patient clean and comfortable. Care for equipment properly.	
___	___	___	20. Perform hand hygiene.	
___	___	___	21. Document the following: amount and type of enema solution used; amount, consistency, and color of stool; pain assessment rating; assessment of perineal area for any irritation, tears, or bleeding; and patient's reaction to procedure.	

Skill Checklists to Accompany Taylor's Clinical Nursing Skills:
A Nursing Process Approach

Name _____ Date _____

Unit _____ Position _____

Instructor/Evaluator: _____ Position _____

SKILL 13-4

Administering a Retention Enema

Goal: To enable patient to expel feces with no evidence of trauma to rectal mucosa.

Excellent	Satisfactory	Needs Practice		Comments
____	____	____	1. Verify the physician's orders, explain the procedure and rationale for the enema to the patient, including where he or she will defecate, and have a bedpan, commode, or nearby bathroom ready for use. Gather equipment. Allow the solution to warm to room temperature	
____	____	____	2. Perform hand hygiene.	
____	____	____	3. Position waterproof pad under the patient.	
____	____	____	4. Provide for patient's privacy. Position and drape the patient on the left side (Sims position) with anus exposed, as dictated by patient comfort and condition.	
____	____	____	5. Put on nonsterile gloves.	
____	____	____	6. Remove cap of prepackaged enema solution and ensure that the rectal tube is prelubricated. If not, apply a generous amount of lubricant to the tube.	
____	____	____	7. Lift the buttock to expose the anus. Slowly and gently insert the rectal tube 7 to 10 cm (3 to 4 inches) Direct it at an angle pointing toward the spine. Ask the patient to take several deep breaths.	
____	____	____	8. If the tube meets resistance while inserting it, permit a small amount of solution to enter, withdraw the tube slightly, and then continue to insert it. Do not force entry of the tube.	
____	____	____	9. Slowly squeeze enema container, emptying entire contents.	
____	____	____	10. Remove while keeping container compressed.	
____	____	____	11. Instruct patient to retain enema solution for at least 30 minutes or as indicated.	
____	____	____	12. Remove nonsterile gloves from inside out and discard.	
____	____	____	13. When the patient has a strong urge to defecate, place him or her in a sitting position on a bedpan or assist to a commode or to the bathroom. Stay with patient or have call light readily accessible.	
____	____	____	14. Remind the patient not to flush commode before nurse inspects results of enema. Record the character of the stool and the patient's reaction to the enema.	

SKILL 13-4
Administering a Retention Enema *(Continued)*

Excellent	Satisfactory	Needs Practice		Comments
___	___	___	15. Assist patient if necessary with cleaning of anal area (putting on gloves if necessary). Offer washcloths, soap, and water to wash patient's hands.	
___	___	___	16. Leave the patient clean and comfortable. Care for the equipment properly.	
___	___	___	17. Perform hand hygiene.	
___	___	___	18. Document the following: amount and type of enema solution used; amount, consistency, and color of stool; pain assessment rating; assessment of perineal area for any irritation, tears, or bleeding; and patient's reaction to procedure.	

Skill Checklists to Accompany Taylor's Clinical Nursing Skills:
A Nursing Process Approach

Name _____ Date _____

Unit _____ Position _____

Instructor/Evaluator: _____ Position _____

Excellent	Satisfactory	Needs Practice	SKILL 13-5 **Administering a Return-Flow Enema (Harris Flush)**	Comments
			Goal: To decrease patient level of pain due to flatus by expelling flatus from rectum.	
___	___	___	1. Verify physician's orders. Explain need for enema to patient, including where he or she will defecate. Have a bedpan, commode, or nearby bathroom ready for use. Gather the necessary equipment.	
___	___	___	2. Warm solution in amount ordered, and check temperature with a bath thermometer if available. (If bath thermometer is not available, warm to room temperature or slightly higher and test on inner wrist.) If tap water is used, adjust temperature as it flows from faucet.	
___	___	___	3. Perform hand hygiene.	
___	___	___	4. Add enema solution to container. Release the clamp and allow fluid to progress through tube before reclamping.	
___	___	___	5. Position waterproof pad under the patient.	
___	___	___	6. Provide for patient's privacy. Position and drape the patient on the left side (Sims position) with anus exposed, as dictated by patient comfort and condition.	
___	___	___	7. Put on nonsterile gloves.	
___	___	___	8. Generously lubricate the end of the rectal tube for 5 to 7 cm (2 to 3 inches) with water-soluble lubricant.	
___	___	___	9. Lift the buttock to expose the anus. Slowly and gently insert the enema tube 7 to 10 cm (3 to 4 inches) Direct it at an angle pointing toward the spine. Ask patient to take several deep breaths.	
___	___	___	10. Elevate the solution so that it flows freely into patient's rectum and sigmoid colon.	
___	___	___	11. If the tube meets resistance while inserting it, permit a small amount of solution to enter, withdraw the tube slightly, and then continue to insert it. Do not force entry of the tube.	
___	___	___	12. After solution has been given, lower container and allow the solution to flow back into container. Repeat this process of allowing solution to flow into rectum and then back into container five or six times.	

Excellent	Satisfactory	Needs Practice	SKILL 13-5 **Administering a Return-Flow Enema** **(Harris Flush)** *(Continued)*	
				Comments
___	___	___	13. If solution becomes thick with feces, replace with fresh solution.	
___	___	___	14. Clamp enema set and remove. Wrap in paper towel.	
___	___	___	15. Allow contaminated solution to flow into toilet and dispose of enema set; if patient feels urge to defecate, assist patient onto bedpan or to the commode.	
___	___	___	16. Assist patient if necessary with cleaning of anal area. Offer washcloths, soap, and water to wash patient's hands.	
___	___	___	17. Remove nonsterile gloves from inside out and discard.	
___	___	___	18. Perform hand hygiene.	
___	___	___	19. Document the following: amount and type of enema solution used; amount, consistency, and color of stool; pain assessment rating; assessment of perineal area for any irritation, tears, or bleeding; changes in abdominal girth or abdominal percussion; and patient's reaction to procedure.	

Skill Checklists to Accompany Taylor's Clinical Nursing Skills:
A Nursing Process Approach

Name _____   Date _____

Unit _____   Position _____

Instructor/Evaluator: _____   Position _____

Excellent	Satisfactory	Needs Practice	SKILL 13-6 **Digital Removal of Stool**	Comments
			Goal: To enable patient to expel feces with assistance.	
——	——	——	1. Verify physician's order; explain procedure to patient, discussing signs and symptoms of a slow heart rate. Instruct patient to report if any of these symptoms are felt during the procedure.	
——	——	——	2. Gather necessary equipment.	
——	——	——	3. Perform hand hygiene.	
——	——	——	4. Place patient in a side-lying position, draping with bath blanket so only buttocks are exposed.	
——	——	——	5. Place waterproof pad under patient's buttocks.	
——	——	——	6. Put on nonsterile gloves.	
——	——	——	7. Generously lubricate the forefinger with water-soluble lubricant and insert the finger gently into the anal canal pointing toward the spine.	
——	——	——	8. Work the finger around and into the hardened mass to break it up and then remove pieces of it. Instruct patient to bear down, if possible, while extracting feces to ease in removal. Place extracted stool in bedpan.	
——	——	——	9. Remove impaction at intervals if it is severe. Instruct patient to alert the nurse if the patient begins to feel lightheaded or nauseated. If patient complains of either symptom, stop removal and assess patient.	
——	——	——	10. Assist patient if necessary with cleaning of anal area. Offer washcloths, soap, and water to wash patient's hands. If patient is able, offer sitz bath.	
——	——	——	11. Remove nonsterile gloves from inside out and discard.	
——	——	——	12. Perform hand hygiene.	
——	——	——	13. Document the following: color, consistency, and amount of stool removed; condition of perianal area after procedure; pain assessment rating; and patient's reaction to procedure.	

Skill Checklists to Accompany Taylor's Clinical Nursing Skills:
A Nursing Process Approach

Name _____   Date _____

Unit _____   Position _____

Instructor/Evaluator: _____   Position _____

Excellent	Satisfactory	Needs Practice	SKILL 13-7 **Applying Fecal Incontinence Pouch**	
			Goal: To enable patient to expel feces into pouch and maintain intact perianal skin.	**Comments**
___	___	___	1. Gather necessary equipment. Discuss reason for fecal incontinence bag with patient	
___	___	___	2. Perform hand hygiene.	
___	___	___	3. Place patient in a side-lying position, draping with bath blanket so only buttocks are exposed.	
___	___	___	4. Put on nonsterile gloves. Cleanse perianal area. Pat dry thoroughly.	
___	___	___	5. Trim perianal hair if needed.	
___	___	___	6. Remove paper backing from adhesive of rectal pouch.	
___	___	___	7. With nondominant hand, separate buttocks. Apply fecal pouch to anal area with dominant hand, ensuring that opening of fecal bag is over anus.	
___	___	___	8. Release buttocks. Attach connector of fecal incontinence pouch to urinary drainage bag. Hang urinary drainage bag below patient.	
___	___	___	9. Remove nonsterile gloves from inside out and discard.	
___	___	___	10. Perform hand hygiene.	
___	___	___	11. Document the following: date and time fecal pouch was applied, appearance of perianal area, color of stool, intake and output (amount of stool), and patient's reaction to procedure.	

Skill Checklists to Accompany Taylor's Clinical Nursing Skills:
A Nursing Process Approach

Name _____   Date _____

Unit _____   Position _____

Instructor/Evaluator: _____   Position _____

Excellent	Satisfactory	Needs Practice	SKILL 13-8 **Changing and Emptying an Ostomy Appliance**	Comments
			Goal: To change and empty ostomy pouch with patient exhibiting no signs and symptoms of peristomal skin breakdown.	
___	___	___	1. Gather the necessary equipment.	
___	___	___	2. Perform hand hygiene and apply nonsterile gloves.	
___	___	___	3. Explain procedure to the patient.	
___	___	___	4. Provide for patient's privacy. Assist to a comfortable sitting or lying position in bed or a standing or sitting position in the bathroom. *To empty a pouch proceed to Action 11. To change a pouch continue with Action 5.*	
___	___	___	5. Empty the partially filled appliance or pouch into a bedpan if it is drainable.	
___	___	___	6. Slowly remove the appliance, beginning at the top while keeping the abdominal skin taut. If any resistance is felt, use warmth or the adhesive solvent to facilitate removal. Discard the disposable appliance or pouch in a plastic bag.	
___	___	___	7. Use toilet tissue to remove any excess stool from the stoma. Cover stoma with a gauze pad. Gently wash and pat dry the peristomal skin. Mild soap may be used to cleanse the peristomal skin, taking care to ensure that all soap is rinsed before reapplying pouch. Do not apply any lotion to the peristomal area.	
___	___	___	8. Assess the appearance of the peristomal skin and stoma. A moist reddish-pink stoma is considered normal.	
___	___	___	9. Apply one-piece or two-piece system:	
___	___	___	a. Select size for stoma opening by using the measurement guide (template).	
___	___	___	b. Trace same size circle on the back and center the skin barrier.	
___	___	___	c. Use scissors to cut an opening ¼ to ⅛ inch larger than stoma.	
___	___	___	d. Remove the backing of protective skin barrier. Apply additional skin protection as necessary.	
___	___	___	e. Remove gauze pad covering stoma.	

Excellent	Satisfactory	Needs Practice	KILL 13-8 **Changing and Emptying an Ostomy Appliance** (*Continued*)	
				Comments
——	——	——	f. Ease barrier and appliance or pouch onto the abdomen and over the stoma, and gently press onto skin while smoothing out creases or wrinkles. Hold in place for 3 minutes.	
——	——	——	10. Close the bottom of appliance or pouch by folding the end upward and using a clamp or clip that comes with product. *Continue to Action 15.*	
			To Empty Appliance or Pouch	
——	——	——	11. Plan to drain the appliance or pouch when it is one-third to one-half full. Remove clamp and fold the end of the pouch upward like a cuff.	
——	——	——	12. Empty contents into bedpan, toilet, or measuring device. Rinse appliance or pouch with tepid water or water mixed with a drop of mouthwash administered with a squeeze bottle.	
——	——	——	13. Wipe the lower 2 inches of the appliance or pouch with toilet tissue.	
——	——	——	14. Uncuff the edge of the appliance or pouch and apply the clip or clamp.	
——	——	——	15. Dispose of used equipment according to agency policy. Remove nonsterile gloves from inside out and discard.	
——	——	——	16. Perform hand hygiene.	
——	——	——	17. Document the following: appearance of stoma, condition of peristomal skin, characteristics of drainage (amount, color, consistency, unusual odor), and patient's reaction to procedure.	

Skill Checklists to Accompany Taylor's Clinical Nursing Skills:
A Nursing Process Approach

Name _____   Date _____

Unit _____   Position _____

Instructor/Evaluator: _____   Position _____

			SKILL 13-9 **Irrigating a Colostomy**	
Excellent	**Satisfactory**	**Needs Practice**	**Goal:** To enable patient to demonstrate ability to participate in care of colostomy.	**Comments**
___	___	___	1. Assemble the necessary equipment. Warm solution in amount ordered. If tap water is used, adjust temperature as it flows from the faucet.	
___	___	___	2. Explain procedure to the patient and plan where he or she will receive irrigation. Assist patient onto bedside commode or into nearby bathroom.	
___	___	___	3. Perform hand hygiene.	
___	___	___	4. Add irrigation solution to container. Release the clamp and allow fluid to progress through the tube before reclamping.	
___	___	___	5. Hang container so that the bottom of bag will be at the patient's shoulder level when seated.	
___	___	___	6. Put on disposable gloves.	
___	___	___	7. Remove appliance and attach irrigation sleeve. Place the drainage end into the toilet bowl or bedpan.	
___	___	___	8. Lubricate the end of the cone with water-soluble lubricant.	
___	___	___	9. Insert the cone into the stoma. Introduce the solution slowly over a period of 5 minutes. Hold tubing (or if patient is able allow patient to hold tubing) all the time that solution is being instilled. Control the rate of flow by closing or opening the clamp.	
___	___	___	10. Hold the cone in place for an additional 10 seconds after the fluid is infused.	
___	___	___	11. Remove the cone. Assist patient to remain seated on toilet or bedside commode.	
___	___	___	12. After most of the solution has returned, allow patient to clip (close) the bottom of the irrigating sleeve and continue with daily activities.	
___	___	___	13. After solution has stopped flowing from stoma, remove irrigating sleeve and cleanse skin around stoma opening with mild soap and water. Gently pat peristomal skin dry.	
___	___	___	14. Attach new appliance to stoma (see Skill 13-8) if needed.	

Excellent	Satisfactory	Needs Practice	SKILL 13-9 **Irrigating a Colostomy** *(Continued)*	
				Comments
___	___	___	15. Document the procedure, including the amount of irrigating solution used; color, amount, and consistency of stool returned; condition of the patient's stoma; degree of patient participation; and patient's reaction to the irrigation.	

Name _____   Date _____

Unit _____   Position _____

Instructor/Evaluator: _____   Position _____

SKILL 13-10

Collecting a Stool Specimen

Goal: To obtain an uncontaminated specimen from patient and send it to the laboratory promptly.

Excellent	Satisfactory	Needs Practice		Comments
___	___	___	1. Gather necessary equipment. Place disposable collection container ("hat") in toilet or bedside commode to catch stool without urine. Explain to patient that he or she should not discard toilet paper with stool and call nurse as soon as bowel movement is completed.	
___	___	___	2. Perform hand hygiene and put on gloves.	
			If Random Stool Collection Is Needed	
___	___	___	3. After the patient has passed a stool, use a clean tongue blade to obtain specimen and place stool in a dry, clean, urine-free container.	
___	___	___	4. Collect as much of the stool as possible to send to the laboratory. If patient is wearing a diaper, the stool may be collected from diaper.	
___	___	___	5. Place lid on container, label with patient's data, and place container in small biohazard bag.	
___	___	___	6. Remove gloves from inside out.	
___	___	___	7. Perform hand hygiene.	
___	___	___	8. Transport to laboratory while stool is still warm. If unable to immediately transport to laboratory, check with laboratory personnel or with policy manual on whether refrigeration is contraindicated.	
			If Stool Is Collected for Ova and Parasites	
___	___	___	9. Follow above steps. Do not refrigerate specimen. Some institutions may require ova and parasite specimens to be placed in container filled with preservatives; check institutional policy.	
___	___	___	10. Document amount, color, and consistency of stool sent.	

Skill Checklists to Accompany Taylor's Clinical Nursing Skills:
A Nursing Process Approach

Name _____   Date _____

Unit _____   Position _____

Instructor/Evaluator: _____   Position _____

Excellent	Satisfactory	Needs Practice	SKILL 14-1 **Using a Pulse Oximeter** **Goal:** To measure oxygen saturation of blood.	Comments
___	___	___	1. Explain procedure to patient.	
___	___	___	2. Perform hand hygiene.	
___	___	___	3. Select an adequate site for application of sensor.	
___	___	___	a. Use patient's index, middle, or ring finger.	
___	___	___	b. Check proximal pulse and capillary refill at pulse closest to site.	
___	___	___	c. If circulation at site is inadequate, an earlobe or bridge of nose may be considered.	
___	___	___	d. Use a toe only if lower extremity circulation is not compromised.	
___	___	___	4. Use the proper equipment.	
___	___	___	a. If one finger is too large for the probe, use a smaller one. A pediatric probe may be used for a small adult.	
___	___	___	b. Use probes appropriate for patient's age and size.	
___	___	___	c. Check if patient is allergic to adhesive. A nonadhesive finger clip or reflectance sensor is available.	
___	___	___	5. Prepare the monitoring site.	
___	___	___	a. Cleanse selected area and allow to dry.	
___	___	___	b. Remove nail polish and artificial nails after checking manufacturer's instructions.	
___	___	___	6. Apply the probe securely to skin. Make sure light-emitting sensor and light-receiving sensor are aligned opposite each other (not necessary to check if placed on forehead or bridge of nose).	
___	___	___	7. Connect sensor probe to pulse oximeter and check operation of equipment (presence of audible beep and fluctuation of bar of light or waveform on the face of the oximeter).	
___	___	___	8. Set alarms on pulse oximeter. Check manufacturer's alarm limits for high and low pulse rate settings.	

Excellent	Satisfactory	Needs Practice	SKILL 14-1 **Using a Pulse Oximeter** *(Continued)*	Comments
___	___	___	9. Check oxygen saturation at regular intervals as ordered by physician and necessitated by alarms. Monitor patient's hemoglobin level.	
___	___	___	10. Remove sensor on a regular basis and check for skin irritation or signs of pressure (every 2 hours for spring-tension sensor or every 4 hours for adhesive finger or toe sensor).	
___	___	___	11. Evaluate any malfunctions or problems with equipment.	
___	___	___	a. For absent or weak signal, check vital signs and patient condition. If satisfactory, check connections and circulation to site.	
___	___	___	b. For inaccurate reading, check prescribed medication and history of circulatory disorders. Try device on a healthy person to see if problem is equipment-related or patient-related.	
___	___	___	c. If bright light (sunlight or fluorescent light) is suspected of causing equipment malfunction, cover probe with a dry washcloth.	
___	___	___	12. Document and report SaO_2 appropriately.	

Skill Checklists to Accompany Taylor's Clinical Nursing Skills:
A Nursing Process Approach

Name _____   Date _____

Unit _____   Position _____

Instructor/Evaluator: _____   Position _____

SKILL 14-2

Teaching Patient to Use an Incentive Spirometer

Excellent	Satisfactory	Needs Practice	**Goal:** To enable the patient to demonstrate increased lung expansion with clear breath sounds.	**Comments**
____	____	____	1. Perform hand hygiene.	
____	____	____	2. Assist patient to an upright or semi-Fowler's position if possible. Remove dentures if poorly fit. Administer pain medication if needed. If patient has recently undergone abdominal surgery, place a pillow over the abdomen for splinting.	
____	____	____	3. Demonstrate how to steady the device with one hand and hold mouthpiece with other hand. If patient is unable to use hands, nurse may assist patient with the incentive spirometer.	
____	____	____	4. Instruct the patient to exhale normally and then place lips securely around the mouthpiece.	
____	____	____	5. Instruct patient to inhale slowly and as deeply as possible through the mouthpiece. Patient should not use nose. If desired a nose clip may be placed.	
____	____	____	6. Tell patient to hold breath and count to 3. Check position of gauge to determine progress and level attained. If patient begins to cough, use pillow to help splint the patient's abdomen.	
____	____	____	7. Instruct patient to remove lips from mouthpiece and exhale normally. Tell patient if he or she becomes lightheaded during the process, stop and take a few normal breaths before resuming incentive spirometer.	
____	____	____	8. Encourage patient to do incentive spirometer 10 times per hour if possible.	
____	____	____	9. Document incentive spirometer done, how many repetitions, and the average volume of the repetitions. If patient coughs, document whether the cough is productive or nonproductive. If the cough is productive, document the consistency, amount, and color of the sputum.	

Name _____   Date _____

Unit _____   Position _____

Instructor/Evaluator: _____   Position _____

Excellent	Satisfactory	Needs Practice	SKILL 14-3 **Instructing Patient to Use a Metered Dose Inhaler**	
			Goal: To teach patient to correctly self-administer medication through an inhaler.	**Comments**
___	___	___	1. Explain procedure to patient.	
___	___	___	2. Perform hand hygiene.	
___	___	___	3. Remove the mouthpiece cover and shake inhaler well.	
			Spacer Technique	
___	___	___	4. Attach the mouthpiece of the inhaler to the spacer.	
___	___	___	5. Instruct the patient to take a deep breath and exhale. Next, have the patient place the spacer's mouthpiece into mouth, grasping securely with teeth and lips, and inhale slowly and deeply through the mouth. Depress the canister (actuator) about one-fourth or one-third of the way through the inspiration.	
			Nonspacer Technique	
___	___	___	6. Have patient hold the inhaler 1 to 2 inches in front of open mouth or have patient place mouthpiece into mouth, grasping it securely with teeth and lips (closed mouth). Instruct the patient to take a deep breath and exhale. Next, have the patient inhale slowly and deeply through the mouth. Press down on the medication canister while continuing to inhale a full breath.	
___	___	___	7. Instruct the patient to hold his or her breath for 5 to 10 seconds or as long as possible and then to exhale slowly through pursed lips.	
___	___	___	8. Wait 1 to 5 minutes before administering the next puff.	
___	___	___	9. After the prescribed amount of puffs have been administered, the patient should remove the spacer (if used) and replace the cap on the mouthpiece.	
___	___	___	10. Reassess lung sounds, oxygenation saturation if ordered, and respirations.	
___	___	___	11. Perform hand hygiene.	
___	___	___	12. Document the patient's respiratory rate, oxygen saturation, and lung sounds.	

Skill Checklists to Accompany Taylor's Clinical Nursing Skills:
A Nursing Process Approach

Name _____   Date _____

Unit _____   Position _____

Instructor/Evaluator: _____   Position _____

Excellent	Satisfactory	Needs Practice	SKILL 14-4 **Administering Medication via a Small Volume Nebulizer** **Goal:** To enable patient to correctly use a nebulizer to self-administer medication.	Comments
___	___	___	1. Explain procedure to patient.	
___	___	___	2. Perform hand hygiene.	
___	___	___	3. Gather equipment. Check physician's order for medication.	
___	___	___	4. Remove the nebulizer cup from the device and open it. Place premeasured unit dose medication in the bottom section of the cup or use a dropper to place concentrated dose of medication in cup and add prescribed fluid to dilute it.	
___	___	___	5. Screw the top portion of nebulizer cup back in place and attach the cup to the nebulizer. Attach one end of tubing to the stem on the bottom of the nebulizer cuff and the other end to the air compressor or oxygen source.	
___	___	___	6. Turn on the air compressor or oxygen. Check that a fine medication mist is produced by opening valve. Place mouthpiece into mouth and grasp securely with teeth and lips.	
___	___	___	7. Instruct the patient to inhale slowly through the mouth (a nose clip may be necessary if patient is also breathing through nose). Hold each breath for 5 to 10 seconds or as long as possible before exhaling.	
___	___	___	8. Continue this inhalation technique until all medication in the nebulizer cup has been aerosolized (usually about 15 minutes). Once the fine mist decreases in amount, gently flick the sides of the nebulizer cup.	
___	___	___	9. If desired, the patient can gargle with tap water after using nebulizer. Rinse the equipment in warm water and allow to air dry on a clean towel.	
___	___	___	10. Reassess lung sounds, oxygenation saturation if ordered, and respirations.	
___	___	___	11. Clean equipment in warm water. Perform hand hygiene.	
___	___	___	12. Document the patient's respiratory rate, oxygen saturation, and lung sounds.	

Skill Checklists to Accompany Taylor's Clinical Nursing Skills:
A Nursing Process Approach

Name _____ Date _____

Unit _____ Position _____

Instructor/Evaluator: _____ Position _____

Excellent	Satisfactory	Needs Practice	SKILL 14-5 **Collecting a Sputum Specimen**	Comments
			Goal: To assist the patient to produce an adequate sample of sputum from the lungs.	
___	___	___	1. Explain procedure to the patient. If patient has pain with coughing, administer pain medication if ordered. If patient can perform task without assistance after instruction, leave container at bedside with instructions to call nurse as soon as specimen is produced.	
___	___	___	2. Assemble equipment.	
___	___	___	3. Perform hand hygiene.	
___	___	___	4. Don disposable gloves and goggles.	
___	___	___	5. Adjust bed to comfortable working position. Lower side rail closer to you. Place the patient in a semi-Fowler's position. Have the patient rinse mouth with water before beginning procedure.	
___	___	___	6. Instruct patient to inhale deeply and cough. If patient has had abdominal surgery, assist patient to splint the abdomen.	
___	___	___	7. If patient produces sputum, open the lid to the container and have patient expectorate specimen into container.	
___	___	___	8. If patient believes they can produce more specimen, have patient repeat the procedure.	
___	___	___	9. Close lid to container. Offer oral hygiene to patient.	
___	___	___	10. Remove gloves. Perform hand hygiene.	
___	___	___	11. Label container with patient's name, time specimen was collected, any antibiotics administered within the last 24 hours, route of collection, and any other information required by institution policy.	
___	___	___	12. Record the time of collecting the specimen, specimen sent, and the nature and amount of secretions. Also note the character of patient's respirations before and after sputum collection. Also note on the laboratory request form any antibiotics administered in the last 24 hours.	

Name _____   Date _____

Unit _____   Position _____

Instructor/Evaluator: _____   Position _____

Excellent	Satisfactory	Needs Practice	SKILL 14-6 **Drawing Arterial Blood Gases**	Comments
			Goal: To obtain blood from the artery without damage to the artery.	
——	——	——	1. Check the patient's identification and confirm the patient's identity. Tell the patient you need to collect an arterial blood sample, and explain the procedure. Tell the patient that the needlestick will cause some discomfort but that he or she must remain still during the procedure. Check the chart to make sure the patient hasn't been suctioned within the past 15 minutes.	
——	——	——	2. Gather equipment and provide privacy. Label the syringe clearly with the patient's name and room number, the physician's name, the date and time of collection, and initials of the person performing the ABG. If not already done, heparinize the syringe and needle:	
——	——	——	a. Attach the 20G needle to the syringe; open the ampule of heparin and withdraw all the heparin into the syringe.	
——	——	——	b. Hold the syringe upright and pull the plunger back slowly to about the 7-mL mark. Rotate the barrel while pulling the plunger back to allow the heparin to coat the inside surface of the syringe. Then slowly force the heparin toward the hub of the syringe and expel all but about 0.1 mL of the heparin.	
——	——	——	c. To heparinize the needle, first replace the 20G needle with the 22G needle. Then hold the syringe upright, tilt it slightly, and eject the remaining heparin.	
——	——	——	3. Perform hand hygiene.	
——	——	——	4. If the patient is on bed rest, ask him or her to lie in a supine position, with the head slightly elevated and the arms at the sides. Ask the ambulatory patient to sit in a chair and support the arm securely on an armrest or a table. Place a waterproof pad under the site and a rolled towel under the wrist.	
——	——	——	5. Perform Allen's test prior to obtaining a specimen from the radial artery:	

Drawing Arterial Blood Gases *(Continued)*

Excellent	Satisfactory	Needs Practice		Comments
—	—	—	a. Have the patient clench the wrist to minimize blood flow into the hand.	
—	—	—	b. Using your index and middle fingers, press on the radial and ulnar arteries. Hold this position for a few seconds.	
—	—	—	c. Without removing your fingers from the arteries, ask the patient to unclench the fist and hold the hand in a relaxed position. The palm will be blanched because pressure from your fingers has impaired the normal blood flow.	
—	—	—	d. Release pressure on the ulnar artery. If the hand becomes flushed, which indicates that blood is filling the vessels, it is safe to proceed with the radial artery puncture. If the hand doesn't flush, perform the test on the other arm.	
—	—	—	6. Perform hand hygiene again and put on gloves.	
—	—	—	7. Locate the radial artery and lightly palpate it for a strong pulse.	
—	—	—	8. Clean the site with an alcohol or povidone–iodine pad (if the patient is not allergic). Don't wipe off the povidone–iodine with alcohol, because alcohol cancels the effect of povidone–iodine. Wipe in a circular motion, spiraling outward from the center of the site. If using alcohol, apply it with friction for 30 seconds or until the final pad comes away clean. Allow the skin to dry.	
—	—	—	9. Stabilize the hand with the wrist extended over the rolled towel. Palpate the artery with the index and middle fingers of one hand while holding the syringe over the puncture site with the other hand. Do not directly touch the area to be stuck.	
—	—	—	10. Hold the needle bevel up at a 45-degree angle at the site of maximal pulse impulse and the shaft parallel to the path of the artery. (When puncturing the brachial artery, hold the needle at a 60-degree angle.)	
—	—	—	11. Puncture the skin and arterial wall in one motion. Watch for blood backflow in the syringe. The pulsating blood will flow into the syringe. Do not pull back on the plunger. Fill the syringe to the 5-mL mark.	
—	—	—	12. After collecting the sample, withdraw the syringe while your nondominant hand is beginning to place pressure proximal to the insertion site with the 2″ × 2″ gauze. Press a gauze pad firmly over the puncture site until the bleeding stops—at least 5 minutes. If the patient is	

			SKILL 14-6

Drawing Arterial Blood Gases (Continued)

Excellent	Satisfactory	Needs Practice		Comments
			receiving anticoagulant therapy or has a blood dyscrasia, apply pressure for 10 to 15 minutes; if necessary, ask a coworker to hold the gauze pad in place while you prepare the sample for transport to the laboratory, but do not ask the patient to hold the pad.	
___	___	___	13. When the bleeding stops, apply a small adhesive bandage or small pressure dressing (fold a 2″ × 2″ gauze into fourths and firmly apply tape, stretching the skin tight).	
___	___	___	14. Once the sample is obtained, check the syringe for air bubbles. If any appear, remove them by holding the syringe upright and slowly ejecting some of the blood onto a 2″ × 2″ gauze pad.	
___	___	___	15. Remove the needle and place the closed cap on the syringe or insert the needle attached to syringe into a rubber stopper. Gently rotate the syringe to ensure that heparin is well distributed. Insert the syringe into a cup or bag of ice.	
___	___	___	16. Attach a properly completed laboratory request form and send the sample to the laboratory immediately.	
___	___	___	17. Remove gloves and perform hand hygiene.	
___	___	___	18. Continue to monitor the patient's vital signs, and monitor the extremity for signs and symptoms such as swelling, discoloration, pain, numbness, or tingling. Watch for bleeding at the puncture site.	
___	___	___	19. Document results of Allen's test, time the sample was drawn, patient's temperature, arterial puncture site, amount of time pressure was applied to the site to control bleeding, type and amount of oxygen therapy, if any, the patient was receiving, pulse oximetry, respiratory rate, and respiratory effort.	

Skill Checklists to Accompany Taylor's Clinical Nursing Skills:
A Nursing Process Approach

Name _____   Date _____

Unit _____   Position _____

Instructor/Evaluator: _____   Position _____

SKILL 14-7

Providing Care of a Chest Tube

Goal: To care for a chest tube without patient experiencing respiratory distress.

Columns: Excellent | Satisfactory | Needs Practice | Comments

1. Explain procedure to patient.
2. Perform hand hygiene and don gloves.
3. Move gown to expose the chest tube insertion site. Observe the dressing around the chest tube insertion site and ensure that it is occlusive. All connections should also be securely taped. Gently palpate around the insertion site, feeling for any subcutaneous emphysema (this will feel crunchy under your fingers).
4. Check drainage tubing to ensure that there are no dependent loops or kinks in the tubing. The drainage collection device must be positioned below the tube insertion site to facilitate drainage.
5. Ensure that a bottle of sterile water or normal saline is at bedside at all times.
6. If the chest tube is ordered to be suctioned, assess the amount of suction set on the chest tube against the amount of suction ordered. Look for any bubbling or tidaling in the suction chamber. The chest tube may be connected to a Heimlich valve, which is one valve to let air out but not in.
7. Measure drainage output at the end of each shift by marking the level on the container or placing a small piece of tape at the drainage level to indicate date and time. The amount should be a running total because the drainage system is never emptied. If the drainage system fills, it will be removed and a new one placed.
8. Obtain two pairs of padded Kelly clamps, new drainage system, and bottle of sterile water. Follow manufacturer's directions to add water to suction system if called for.
9. Apply Kelly clamps 1½ to 2½ inches from insertion site and 1 inch apart, going in opposite directions.
10. Prepare new drainage system. Don disposable gloves.

Excellent	Satisfactory	Needs Practice		Comments
——	——	——	11. Remove the suction from the drainage system. Use scissors to cut away any foam tape on connection of chest tube and drainage system. Using a slight twisting motion, remove the drainage system. Do not pull on the chest tube.	
——	——	——	12. Keeping end of chest tube sterile, insert end of new drainage system into chest tube. Reconnect suction if ordered. Apply plastic bands or foam tape to chest tube/drainage system connection site. Remove Kelly clamps.	
——	——	——	13. Assess drainage system for continuous bubbling, tidaling, and amount of suction applied.	
——	——	——	14. Remove gloves. Perform hand hygiene.	
——	——	——	15. Document the site of the chest tube, amount and type of drainage, amount of suction applied, and any bubbling, tidaling, or subcutaneous emphysema noted. Document the type of dressing in place and the patient's pain response as well as any measures done to relieve the patient's pain.	

Name _____ Date _____

Unit _____ Position _____

Instructor/Evaluator: _____ Position _____

Excellent	Satisfactory	Needs Practice	SKILL 14-8 **Assisting with Removal of a Chest Tube**	
			Goal: To assist with removal or a chest tube while keeping patient free of respiratory distress.	**Comments**
___	___	___	1. Explain procedure to patient.	
___	___	___	2. Perform hand hygiene.	
___	___	___	3. Administer pain medication.	
___	___	___	4. Don gloves.	
___	___	___	5. Provide reassurance to patient while physician removes dressing.	
___	___	___	6. After physician has removed chest tube and secured occlusive dressing, assess patient's lung sounds, respiratory rate, oxygen saturation, and pain level.	
___	___	___	7. Anticipate the physician ordering a chest x-ray.	
___	___	___	8. Dispose of equipment appropriately. Remove gloves and dispose. Perform hand hygiene.	
___	___	___	9. Document the patient's respiratory rate, oxygen saturation, lung sounds, total of chest tube output, and status of dressing.	

Skill Checklists to Accompany Taylor's Clinical Nursing Skills:
A Nursing Process Approach

Name _____   Date _____

Unit _____   Position _____

Instructor/Evaluator: _____   Position _____

Excellent	Satisfactory	Needs Practice	SKILL 14-9 **Administering Oxygen by Nasal Cannula** **Goal:** To provide oxygen delivery via nasal cannula; patient oxygen saturation level will be within acceptable parameters.	**Comments**
____	____	____	1. Explain procedure to patient and review safety precautions necessary when oxygen is in use. Place No Smoking signs in appropriate areas.	
____	____	____	2. Perform hand hygiene.	
____	____	____	3. Connect nasal cannula to oxygen setup with humidification, if one is in use. Adjust flow rate as ordered by physician. Check that oxygen is flowing out of prongs.	
____	____	____	4. Place the prongs in patient's nostrils. Adjust according to type of equipment.	
____	____	____	a. Over and behind each ear with adjuster comfortably under chin; or	
____	____	____	b. Around patient's head.	
____	____	____	5. Use gauze pads at ear beneath tubing as necessary. Adjust cannula as necessary.	
____	____	____	6. Encourage patient to breathe through nose with mouth closed.	
____	____	____	7. Perform hand hygiene.	
____	____	____	8. Assess and chart patient's response to therapy.	
____	____	____	9. Remove and clean cannula and assess nares at least every 8 hours or according to agency recommendations. Check nares for evidence of irritation or bleeding.	
____	____	____	10. Document the amount of oxygen applied, the patient's respiratory rate, oxygen saturation, and lung sounds.	

Skill Checklists to Accompany Taylor's Clinical Nursing Skills:
A Nursing Process Approach

Name _____ Date _____

Unit _____ Position _____

Instructor/Evaluator: _____ Position _____

SKILL 14-10

Administering Oxygen by Mask

Goal: To provide oxygen delivery via a mask apparatus; patient exhibits an oxygen saturation within acceptable parameters.

Excellent	Satisfactory	Needs Practice		Comments
___	___	___	1. Explain procedure to patient and review safety precautions necessary when oxygen is in use. Place No Smoking signs in appropriate areas.	
___	___	___	2. Perform hand hygiene.	
___	___	___	3. Attach face mask to oxygen setup with humidification. Start flow of oxygen at specified rate. For a mask with a reservoir, allow oxygen to fill bag before placing mask over patient's nose and mouth.	
___	___	___	4. Position face mask over patient's nose and mouth. Adjust it with the elastic strap so mask fits snugly but comfortably on face. Adjust the flow rate.	
___	___	___	5. Use gauze pads to reduce irritation on patient's ears and scalp.	
___	___	___	6. Perform hand hygiene.	
___	___	___	7. Remove mask and dry skin every 2 to 3 hours if oxygen is running continuously. Do not powder around mask.	
___	___	___	8. Assess and chart patient's response to therapy.	
___	___	___	9. Document the type of mask used, the amount of oxygen used, the oxygen saturation, the lung sounds, and the rate/pattern of respirations.	

Skill Checklists to Accompany Taylor's Clinical Nursing Skills:
A Nursing Process Approach

Name _____   Date _____

Unit _____   Position _____

Instructor/Evaluator: _____   Position _____

SKILL 14-11
Using an Oxygen Hood

Excellent	Satisfactory	Needs Practice	**Goal:** To deliver oxygen via hood; patient exhibits an oxygen saturation within acceptable parameters.	Comments
——	——	——	1. Explain procedure to patient and review safety precautions necessary when oxygen is in use. Place No Smoking signs in appropriate areas.	
——	——	——	2. Perform hand hygiene.	
——	——	——	3. Place hood on crib. Connect the humidifier to the oxygen source in the wall. Insert oxygen tubing from humidifier into hole on the back of the oxygen hood. Adjust the flow rate as ordered by physician. Check that oxygen is flowing into hood.	
——	——	——	4. Turn analyzer on. Place oxygen analyzer probe in the crib.	
——	——	——	5. Adjust oxygen flow as necessary. Once oxygen levels reach the prescribed amount, place hood over patient's head.	
——	——	——	6. If using the soft vinyl hood, roll small blankets or towels and place around edges where hood meets crib if needed to keep oxygen concentration at desired level. Do not block hole in top of hood if present. If using the vinyl hoods, the hole covering may need to be removed.	
——	——	——	7. Encourage family members not to raise edges of the hood.	
——	——	——	8. Frequently check bedding and patient's head for moisture.	
——	——	——	9. Perform hand hygiene.	
——	——	——	10. Document the amount of oxygen applied and the patient's respiratory rate, oxygen saturation, and lung sounds.	

Name _____   Date _____

Unit _____   Position _____

Instructor/Evaluator: _____   Position _____

			SKILL 14-12	
Excellent	**Satisfactory**	**Needs Practice**	**Using an Oxygen Tent**	
			Goal: To administer oxygen via tent; patient exhibits an oxygen saturation within acceptable parameters.	**Comments**
___	___	___	1. Explain procedure to patient and review safety precautions necessary when oxygen is in use. Place No Smoking signs in appropriate areas.	
___	___	___	2. Perform hand hygiene.	
___	___	___	3. Place tent over crib or bed. Connect the humidifier to the oxygen source in the wall. Insert oxygen tubing connected to the humidifier inside the tent out of the patient's reach. Adjust the flow rate as ordered by physician. Check that oxygen is flowing into tent.	
___	___	___	4. Turn analyzer on. Place oxygen analyzer probe in the tent out of the patient's reach.	
___	___	___	5. Adjust oxygen as necessary. Once oxygen levels reach the prescribed amount, place patient in the bed.	
___	___	___	6. Tuck tent edges under blanket.	
___	___	___	7. Encourage patient and family members to keep tent flap closed.	
___	___	___	8. Frequently check bedding and patient's pajamas for moisture.	
___	___	___	9. Perform hand hygiene.	
___	___	___	10. Document the amount of oxygen applied and the patient's respiratory rate, oxygen saturation, and lung sounds.	

Skill Checklists to Accompany Taylor's Clinical Nursing Skills:
A Nursing Process Approach

Name _____ Date _____

Unit _____ Position _____

Instructor/Evaluator: _____ Position _____

SKILL 14-13
Inserting an Oropharyngeal Airway

Goal: To insert a patent oral airway.

Excellent	Satisfactory	Needs Practice		Comments
___	___	___	1. Gather equipment. Explain procedure to patient and patient's family.	
___	___	___	2. Perform hand hygiene.	
___	___	___	3. Measure the oropharyngeal airway for correct size.	
___	___	___	4. Don disposable gloves.	
___	___	___	5. Check the patient's mouth for any loose teeth, candy, or dentures.	
___	___	___	6. Position patient on his or her back with neck hyperextended (unless this is contraindicated).	
___	___	___	7. Open patient's mouth by using your thumb and index finger to gently pry teeth apart. Insert the airway with the curved tip pointing up toward the roof of the mouth.	
___	___	___	8. Slide the airway across the tongue to the back of the mouth. Rotate the airway 180 degrees as it passes the uvula (a flashlight can confirm the position of the airway with the curve fitting over the tongue).	
___	___	___	9. Ensure accurate placement and adequate ventilation by auscultating breath sounds.	
___	___	___	10. Position patient on his or her side when airway is in place.	
___	___	___	11. Remove the airway for a brief period every 4 hours. Provide mouth care and rinse airway before reinserting it.	
___	___	___	12. Remove gloves and perform hand hygiene.	
___	___	___	13. Document the placement of the airway as well as lung sounds and pulse oximetry.	

Skill Checklists to Accompany Taylor's Clinical Nursing Skills:
A Nursing Process Approach

Name _____   Date _____

Unit _____   Position _____

Instructor/Evaluator: _____   Position _____

SKILL 14-14

Suctioning Nasopharyngeal and Oropharyngeal Airways

Goal: To remove secretions from oropharyngeal and nasopharyngeal airways.

Excellent	Satisfactory	Needs Practice		Comments
___	___	___	1. Determine need for suctioning. Administer pain medication before suctioning to postoperative patient.	
___	___	___	2. Explain procedure to patient.	
___	___	___	3. Assemble equipment.	
___	___	___	4. Perform hand hygiene.	
___	___	___	5. Adjust bed to comfortable working position. Lower side rail closer to you. Place patient in a semi-Fowler's position if he or she is conscious. An unconscious patient should be placed in the lateral position facing you.	
___	___	___	6. Place towel or waterproof pad across patient's chest.	
___	___	___	7. Turn suction to appropriate pressure.	
___	___	___	a. Wall unit: Adult: 100 to 120 mm Hg	
			b. Portable unit: Adult: 10 to 15 cm Hg	
___	___	___	8. Open sterile suction package. Set up sterile container, touching only the outside surface, and pour sterile saline into it.	
___	___	___	9. Don sterile gloves. The dominant hand that will handle catheter must remain sterile, whereas the nondominant hand is considered clean rather than sterile.	
___	___	___	10. With sterile gloved hand, pick up sterile catheter and connect to suction tubing held with unsterile hand.	
___	___	___	11. Moisten catheter by dipping it into container of sterile saline. Occlude Y-tube to check suction.	
___	___	___	12. Estimate the distance from earlobe to nostril and place thumb and forefinger of gloved hand at that point on catheter.	
___	___	___	13. Gently insert catheter with suction off by leaving the vent on the Y-connector open. Slip catheter gently along the floor of an unobstructed nostril toward trachea to suction the nasopharynx. Or insert catheter along side of mouth	

Suctioning Nasopharyngeal and Oropharyngeal Airways *(Continued)*

Excellent	Satisfactory	Needs Practice		Comments
			toward trachea to suction the oropharynx. Never apply suction as catheter is introduced.	
___	___	___	14. Apply suction intermittently by occluding suctioning port with your thumb. Gently rotate catheter as it is being withdrawn. Do not allow suctioning to continue for more than 10 to 15 seconds at a time.	
___	___	___	15. Flush the catheter with saline and repeat suctioning as needed and according to patient's toleration of the procedure.	
___	___	___	16. Allow at least a 20- to 30-second interval if additional suctioning is needed. The nares should be alternated when repeated suctioning is required. Do not force the catheter through the nares. Encourage patient to cough and breathe deeply between suctionings. Suction the oropharynx.	
___	___	___	17. When suctioning is completed, remove gloves inside out and dispose of gloves, catheter, and container with solution in proper receptacle. Perform hand hygiene.	
___	___	___	18. Use auscultation to listen to chest and breath sounds to assess effectiveness of suctioning.	
___	___	___	19. Record time of suctioning and nature and amount of secretions. Also note the character of the patient's respirations before and after suctioning.	
___	___	___	20. Offer oral hygiene after suctionings.	

Skill Checklists to Accompany Taylor's Clinical Nursing Skills:
A Nursing Process Approach

Name _____ Date _____

Unit _____ Position _____

Instructor/Evaluator: _____ Position _____

Excellent	Satisfactory	Needs Practice	SKILL 14-15 **Inserting a Nasal Airway**	
			Goal: To sustain and maintain a patent airway.	**Comments**
___	___	___	1. Gather equipment. Explain procedure to patient.	
___	___	___	2. Perform hand hygiene.	
___	___	___	3. Measure the nasopharyngeal airway for correct size.	
___	___	___	4. Don disposable gloves. If patient is coughing or has copious secretions, a mask and goggles may also be worn.	
___	___	___	5. Adjust bed to a comfortable working level. Lower the side rail closer to you. If patient is awake and alert, position patient supine in semi-Fowler's position. If patient is not conscious or alert, position patient in a side-lying position.	
___	___	___	6. Lubricate the nasopharyngeal airway generously with a water-soluble lubricant, covering the airway from the tip to the guard rim.	
___	___	___	7. Gently insert the airway into the naris until the rim is touching the naris. If resistance is met, stop and try other naris.	
___	___	___	8. Remove the airway and place in other naris at least every 24 hours.	
___	___	___	9. If patient needs to be suctioned, follow steps in Skill 14-14. Ensure that suction catheter is lubricated with water before suctioning to prevent any trauma to mucosa. Document the placement of the nasopharyngeal airway including: size of airway, naris placed in, and respiratory status before and after placement.	

Skill Checklists to Accompany Taylor's Clinical Nursing Skills:
A Nursing Process Approach

Name _____   Date _____

Unit _____   Position _____

Instructor/Evaluator: _____   Position _____

Excellent	Satisfactory	Needs Practice	SKILL 14-16 **Suctioning the Tracheostomy**	Comments
			Goal: To remove secretions from an artificial airway and promote oxygen exchange.	
____	____	____	1. Explain the procedure to the patient and reassure him or her that you will interrupt the procedure if the patient indicates respiratory difficulty. Administer pain medication to postoperative patient before suctioning.	
____	____	____	2. Gather equipment and provide privacy for patient.	
____	____	____	3. Perform hand hygiene.	
____	____	____	4. Assist the patient to a semi-Fowler's or Fowler's position if conscious. An unconscious patient should be placed in the lateral position facing you.	
____	____	____	5. Turn suction to appropriate pressure.	
____	____	____	a. Wall unit: Adult: 100 to 120 mm Hg	
____	____	____	b. Portable unit: Adult: 10 to 15 cm Hg	
____	____	____	6. Place clean towel, if being used, across patient's chest. Don goggles, mask, and gown, if necessary.	
____	____	____	7. Open sterile kit or set up equipment and prepare to suction.	
____	____	____	a. Place sterile drape, if available, across patient's chest.	
____	____	____	b. Open sterile container and place on bedside table or overbed table without contaminating inner surface. Pour sterile saline into it.	
____	____	____	c. Hyperoxygenate patient using manual resuscitation bag or sigh mechanism on mechanical ventilator.	
____	____	____	d. Don sterile gloves or one sterile glove on dominant hand and clean glove on nondominant hand.	
____	____	____	e. Connect sterile suction catheter to suction tubing held with unsterile gloved hand.	
____	____	____	8. Holding catheter with sterile dominant hand, moisten by dipping it into the container of sterile saline, unless it is one of the newer silicone catheters that does not require lubrication. Check suction on catheter by occluding the Y-port.	

Suctioning the Tracheostomy *(Continued)*

Excellent	Satisfactory	Needs Practice		Comments
___	___	___	9. Remove oxygen delivery setup with unsterile gloved hand if it is still in place.	
___	___	___	10. Using sterile gloved hand, gently and quickly insert catheter into the trachea. Advance about 10 to 12. 5 cm (4 to 5 inches) or until patient coughs. Do not occlude Y-port when inserting catheter.	
___	___	___	11. Apply intermittent suction by occluding Y-port with thumb of unsterile gloved hand. Gently rotate catheter with thumb and index finger of sterile gloved hand as catheter is being withdrawn. Do not allow suctioning to continue for more than 10 seconds. Hyperventilate three to five times between suctionings or encourage patient to cough and breathe deeply between suctionings.	
___	___	___	12. Flush catheter with saline and repeat suctioning as needed and according to patient's tolerance of the procedure. Allow patient to rest at least 1 minute between suctionings and replace oxygen delivery setup if necessary. Limit suctioning events to three times.	
___	___	___	13. When procedure is completed, turn off suction and disconnect catheter from suction tubing. Remove gloves inside out and dispose of gloves, catheter, and container with solution in proper receptacle. Perform hand hygiene.	
___	___	___	14. Adjust patient's position. Reapply patient's oxygen supply if indicated. Auscultate chest to evaluate breath sounds.	
___	___	___	15. Record time of suctioning and nature and amount of secretions. Also note character of patient's respirations before and after suctioning.	
___	___	___	16. Offer oral hygiene.	

Skill Checklists to Accompany Taylor's Clinical Nursing Skills:
A Nursing Process Approach

Name _____ Date _____

Unit _____ Position _____

Instructor/Evaluator: _____ Position _____

SKILL 14-17
Providing Tracheostomy Care

Goal: To clean artificial airway and prevent accumulation of secretions that interfere with oxygenation.

Excellent	Satisfactory	Needs Practice		Comments
___	___	___	1. Explain procedure to patient.	
___	___	___	2. If tracheostomy tube has just been suctioned, remove soiled dressing from around tube and discard with gloves on removal.	
___	___	___	3. Perform hand hygiene and open necessary supplies.	
			Cleaning a Nondisposable Inner Cannula	
___	___	___	4. Prepare supplies before cleaning inner cannula.	
___	___	___	a. Open tracheostomy care kit and separate basins, touching only the edges. If kit is not available, open two sterile basins.	
___	___	___	b. Fill one basin ½ inch (1.25 cm) deep with hydrogen peroxide.	
___	___	___	c. Fill other basin ½ inch (1.25 cm) deep with saline.	
___	___	___	d. Open sterile brush or pipe cleaners if they are not already in cleaning kit. Open additional sterile gauze pad.	
___	___	___	5. Don disposable gloves.	
___	___	___	6. Remove oxygen source if one is present. Rotate lock on inner cannula in a counterclockwise motion to release it.	
___	___	___	7. Gently remove inner cannula and carefully drop it in basin with hydrogen peroxide. Remove gloves and discard.	
___	___	___	8. Clean inner cannula.	
___	___	___	a. Don sterile gloves.	
___	___	___	b. Remove inner cannula from soaking solution. Moisten brush or pipe cleaners in saline and insert into tube, using back-and-forth motion.	
___	___	___	c. Agitate cannula in saline solution. Remove and tap against inner surface of basin.	
___	___	___	d. Place on sterile gauze pad.	
___	___	___	9. Suction outer cannula using sterile technique if necessary.	

Skill 14-17

Providing Tracheostomy Care *(Continued)*

Excellent	Satisfactory	Needs Practice		Comments
—	—	—	10. Replace inner cannula into outer cannula. Turn lock clockwise and make sure that inner cannula is secure. Reapply oxygen source if needed.	
			Replacing Disposable Inner Cannula	
—	—	—	11. Release lock. Gently remove inner cannula and place in disposable bag. Discard gloves and don sterile ones to insert new cannula. Replace with appropriately sized new cannula. Engage lock on inner cannula.	
			Applying Clean Dressing and Tape	
—	—	—	12. Dip cotton-tipped applicator in sterile saline and clean stoma under faceplate. Use each applicator only once, moving from stoma site outward.	
—	—	—	13. If secretions prove difficult to remove, apply diluted ½ strength hydrogen peroxide to area around stoma, faceplate, and outer cannula. Rinse area with saline.	
—	—	—	14. Pat skin gently with dry 4″ × 4″ gauze.	
—	—	—	15. Slide commercially prepared tracheostomy dressing or prefolded noncotton-filled 4″ × 4″ dressing under faceplate.	
—	—	—	16. Change tracheostomy tape.	
—	—	—	a. Leave soiled tape in place until new one is applied.	
—	—	—	b. Cut piece of tape that is twice the neck circumference plus 4 inches (10 cm). Trim ends on the diagonal.	
—	—	—	c. Insert one end of tape through faceplate opening alongside old tape. Pull through until both ends are even.	
—	—	—	d. Slide both tapes under patient's neck and insert one end through remaining opening on other side of faceplate. Pull snugly and tie ends in double square knot. Check that patient can flex neck comfortably.	
—	—	—	e. Carefully remove old tape. Reapply oxygen source if necessary.	
—	—	—	17. Remove gloves and discard. Perform hand hygiene. Assess patient's respirations. Document assessments and completion of procedure.	

Skill Checklists to Accompany Taylor's Clinical Nursing Skills:
A Nursing Process Approach

Name _____   Date _____

Unit _____   Position _____

Instructor/Evaluator: _____   Position _____

Excellent	Satisfactory	Needs Practice	SKILL 14-18 **Retaping an Endotracheal Tube**	
			Goal: To keep patient's tube in place with patient having bilaterally equal and clear lung sounds.	**Comments**
____	____	____	1. Explain procedure to patient and reassure him or her that you will interrupt procedure if the patient indicates respiratory difficulty. Administer pain medication and or sedation before attempting to retape endotracheal tube.	
____	____	____	2. Gather equipment and provide privacy for patient.	
____	____	____	3. Perform hand hygiene.	
____	____	____	4. Suction patient as previous described in Skill 14-16.	
____	____	____	5. Cut tape. Use enough tape to go around patient's neck to the mouth plus 8 inches.	
____	____	____	6. Cut another piece of tape long enough to reach from one jaw, around the backside of the neck to the other jaw. Match the tapes' adhesive sides together in the center of the longer piece of tape.	
____	____	____	7. Take one 3-mL syringe and wrap the sticky tape around the syringe until the nonsticky area is reached. Do this for the other side as well.	
____	____	____	8. Take one of the 3-mL syringes and pass it under the patient's neck so that there is a 3-mL syringe on either side of the patient's head.	
____	____	____	9. Don disposable gloves. (Have assistant don gloves as well.)	
____	____	____	10. Provide oral care, including suctioning the oral cavity.	
____	____	____	11. Begin to unwrap old tape from around the endotracheal tube. After one side is unwrapped, have assistant hold tube to offer stabilization. Instruct assistant to hold tube as close to the lips or nares as possible.	
____	____	____	12. After tape is removed, have assistant gently and slowly move endotracheal tube (if orally intubated) to the other side of the mouth. Assess mouth for any skin breakdown. Before applying new tape, make sure that markings on endotracheal tube are at same spot as when retaping began.	

Excellent	Satisfactory	Needs Practice	SKILL 14-18 **Retaping an Endotracheal Tube** *(Continued)*	
				Comments
____	____	____	13. Remove old tape from cheeks and side of face. Wash area to remove old tape and benzoin. If patient is male, consider shaving cheeks. Pat cheeks dry with a 4″ × 4″ gauze.	
____	____	____	14. Consider applying benzoin. Unroll one side of the tape. Ensure that nonsticky part of tape remains behind patient's neck while pulling firmly on the tape. Place adhesive portion of tape snugly against patient's cheek. Split the tape in half from the end to the corner of the mouth.	
____	____	____	15. Wrap the top half-piece of split tape around the tube in one direction and then secure it across the upper lip. Wrap the bottom half-piece around the endotracheal tube in the opposite direction and secure the tape beneath the lower lip. Fold over tab on end of tape.	
____	____	____	16. Unwrap second piece of tape. Split to corner of the mouth. Reversing the order, place bottom piece of tape on the top lip. Wrap top piece of tape in a counterclockwise manner and secure to the lower lip. Fold over tab on end of tape.	
____	____	____	17. Auscultate lung sounds. Assess for cyanosis, oxygen saturation, chest symmetry, and stableness of endotracheal tube. Again check to ensure that the tube is at the correct depth.	
____	____	____	18. If endotracheal tube is cuffed, check pressure of balloon by attaching a hand-held pressure gauge to the pilot balloon of the endotracheal tube.	
____	____	____	19. Remove gloves and perform hand hygiene.	
____	____	____	20. Document the procedure, including the depth of the endotracheal tube from teeth or lips; amount, consistency, and color of secretions suctioned; presence of any pressure ulcers; lung sounds; oxygen saturation; skin color; cuff pressure; and chest symmetry.	

Skill Checklists to Accompany Taylor's Clinical Nursing Skills: A Nursing Process Approach

Name _____   Date _____

Unit _____   Position _____

Instructor/Evaluator: _____   Position _____

SKILL 14-19
Suctioning an Endotracheal Tube

Goal: To maintain a patent airway.

Excellent	Satisfactory	Needs Practice		Comments
___	___	___	**Open System Suctioning**	
			1. Explain procedure to patient and reassure him or her that you will interrupt procedure if the patient indicates respiratory difficulty. Administer pain medication before suctioning to postoperative patient.	
___	___	___	2. Gather equipment and provide privacy for patient.	
___	___	___	3. Perform hand hygiene.	
___	___	___	4. Assist the patient to a semi-Fowler's or Fowler's position.	
___	___	___	5. Turn suction to appropriate pressure.	
___	___	___	6. Place clean towel, if being used, across patient's chest. Don goggles, mask, and gown, if necessary.	
___	___	___	7. Open sterile kit or set up equipment and prepare to suction.	
___	___	___	a. Place sterile drape, if available, across patient's chest.	
___	___	___	b. Open sterile container and place on bedside table or overbed table without contaminating inner surface. Pour sterile saline into it.	
___	___	___	c. Hyperoxygenate patient using manual resuscitation bag (may be easier to have assistant deliver breaths) or sigh mechanism on ventilator.	
___	___	___	d. Don sterile gloves or one sterile glove on dominant hand and clean glove on nondominant hand.	
___	___	___	e. Connect sterile suction catheter to suction tubing that is held with unsterile gloved hand.	
___	___	___	8. Keeping catheter wrapped around sterile hand, remove ventilator from endotracheal tube with nonsterile hand.	
___	___	___	9. Hyperoxygenate or hyperventilate with manual resuscitation bag three to five times between suctionings. Keeping the catheter sterile, gently insert the catheter into the endotracheal tube, advancing until patient begins to cough or resistance is met. Do not occlude Y port when inserting catheter.	

Excellent	Satisfactory	Needs Practice		Comments

Suctioning an Endotracheal Tube *(Continued)*

Excellent	Satisfactory	Needs Practice		Comments
___	___	___	10. Apply intermittent suction by occluding Y port with thumb of unsterile gloved hand. Gently rotate catheter with thumb and index finger of sterile gloved hand as catheter is being withdrawn. Do not allow suctioning to continue for more than 10 seconds.	
___	___	___	11. Flush the catheter with saline and repeat suctioning as needed and according to patient's toleration of procedure. Allow patient to rest at least 1 minute between suctionings and replace oxygen delivery setup if necessary. Limit suctioning events to three times. Reconnect to the ventilator and hyperoxygenate or hyperventilate with manual resuscitation bag three to five times between suctionings.	
___	___	___	12. When procedure is completed, turn off suction and disconnect catheter from suction tubing. Remove gloves inside out and dispose of gloves, catheter, and container with solution in proper receptacle.	
___	___	___	13. Suction the oral cavity and perform oral hygiene.	
___	___	___	14. Perform hand hygiene.	
___	___	___	15. Adjust patient's position. Auscultate chest to evaluate breath sounds.	
___	___	___	16. Record the time of suctioning and the nature and amount of secretions. Also note the character of patient's respirations before and after suctioning.	

Closed System Suctioning

Excellent	Satisfactory	Needs Practice		Comments
___	___	___	1. Explain procedure to patient and reassure him or her that you will interrupt procedure if the patient indicates respiratory difficulty. Administer pain medication before suctioning to postoperative patient.	
___	___	___	2. Gather equipment and provide privacy for patient.	
___	___	___	3. Perform hand hygiene.	
___	___	___	4. Assist the patient to a semi-Fowler's or Fowler's position.	

To Use a Closed Suction Device

Excellent	Satisfactory	Needs Practice		Comments
___	___	___	5. Open sterile package of closed suction device. Make sure that the device remains sterile.	
___	___	___	6. Don sterile gloves.	
___	___	___	7. Using nondominant hand, disconnect the ventilator from the endotracheal tube. Place ventilator tubing so that the inside of the tubing remains sterile.	

SKILL 14-19
Suctioning an Endotracheal Tube *(Continued)*

Excellent	Satisfactory	Needs Practice		Comments
___	___	___	8. Using dominant hand and keeping device sterile, connect the closed suctioning device so that suctioning catheter is parallel with the endotracheal tube. Attach suction tubing to suction catheter (do not need to remain sterile for this step).	
___	___	___	9. Keeping inside of the ventilator tubing sterile, attach ventilator tubing to port perpendicular to the endotracheal tube.	
___	___	___	10. Turn suction to appropriate pressure.	
___	___	___	11. Pop top off of sterile normal saline dosette. Open plug to port by suction catheter and insert saline dosette.	
___	___	___	12. Hyperoxygenate or hyperventilate by using the sigh button on the ventilator before suctioning. Turn safety cap on suction button of catheter so that button is easily depressed.	
___	___	___	13. Grasp suction catheter through protective sheath, about 6 inches (15 cm) from endotracheal tube. Gently insert the catheter into the endotracheal tube. Release the catheter while holding onto the protective sheath. Return sheath to original place. Grasp catheter through sheath and repeat procedure advancing until patient begins to cough. Do not occlude Y port when inserting catheter.	
___	___	___	14. Apply intermittent suction by depressing the suction button with thumb of nondominant hand. Gently rotate catheter with thumb and index finger of dominant hand as catheter is being withdrawn. Do not allow suctioning to continue for more than 10 seconds. Hyperoxygenate or hyperventilate with sigh button on ventilator as ordered.	
___	___	___	15. Once catheter is withdrawn back into sheath, depress the suction button while gently squeezing the normal saline dosette until catheter is clean. Allow patient to rest at least 1 minute between suctionings and replace oxygen delivery setup if necessary. Limit suctioning events to three times.	
___	___	___	16. When procedure is completed, ensure that catheter is withdrawn into sheath and turn safety button. Remove normal saline dosette and apply cap to port.	
___	___	___	17. Suction the oral cavity and perform oral hygiene.	
___	___	___	18. Perform hand hygiene.	
___	___	___	19. Adjust patient's position. Auscultate chest to evaluate breath sounds.	

Excellent	Satisfactory	Needs Practice	SKILL 14-19 **Suctioning an Endotracheal Tube** *(Continued)*	Comments
___	___	___	20. Record the time of suctioning and the nature and amount of secretions. Also note the character of patient's respirations before and after suctioning.	

Skill Checklists to Accompany Taylor's Clinical Nursing Skills:
A Nursing Process Approach

Name _____   Date _____

Unit _____   Position _____

Instructor/Evaluator: _____   Position _____

Excellent	Satisfactory	Needs Practice	SKILL 14-20 **Collecting a Sputum Specimen via Suctioning (Endotracheal Tube)**	
			Goal: To gain a sputum specimen while airway patency is maintained.	**Comments**
—— —— ——			1. Explain procedure to patient and reassure him or her that you will interrupt procedure if the patient indicates respiratory difficulty. Administer pain medication before suctioning to postoperative patient.	
—— —— ——			2. Gather equipment and provide privacy for patient.	
—— —— ——			3. Perform hand hygiene.	
—— —— ——			4. Assist the patient to a semi-Fowler's or Fowler's position.	
—— —— ——			5. Connect specimen container to suction tubing. Turn suction to appropriate pressure.	
—— —— ——			6. Place clean towel, if being used, across patient's chest. Don goggles, mask, and gown, if necessary.	
—— —— ——			7. Open sterile kit or set up equipment and prepare to suction.	
—— —— ——			a. Place sterile drape, if available, across patient's chest.	
—— —— ——			b. Open sterile container and place on bedside table or overbed table without contaminating inner surface. Pour sterile saline into it.	
—— —— ——			c. Hyperoxygenate patient using manual resuscitation bag (may be easier if assistant delivers breaths with bag) or sigh mechanism on ventilator.	
—— —— ——			d. Don sterile gloves or one sterile glove on dominant hand and clean glove on nondominant hand.	
—— —— ——			e. Connect sterile suction catheter to specimen container that is held with unsterile gloved hand.	
—— —— ——			8. Keeping catheter wrapped around sterile hand, remove ventilator from endotracheal tube with nonsterile hand.	
—— —— ——			9. Hyperoxygenate or hyperventilate with manual resuscitation bag three to five times between suctionings. Keeping the catheter sterile, gently insert the catheter into the endotracheal tube advancing until resistance is met or the patient begins to cough. Do not occlude Y port when inserting catheter.	

Excellent	Satisfactory	Needs Practice	SKILL 14-20 **Collecting a Sputum Specimen via Suctioning** **(Endotracheal Tube)** *(Continued)*	
				Comments
___	___	___	10. Apply intermittent suction by occluding Y port with thumb of unsterile gloved hand. Gently rotate catheter with thumb and index finger of sterile gloved hand as catheter is being withdrawn. Do not allow suctioning to continue for more than 10 seconds. Reconnect to the ventilator and hyperoxygenate or hyperventilate with manual resuscitation bag three to five times between suctionings.	
___	___	___	11. Repeat suctioning as needed and according to patient's toleration of procedure. If 1 to 2 mL of sputum has been obtained, disconnect specimen container and connect suction tubing to the suction catheter. The catheter may then be flushed with normal saline before repeat suctioning. If less than 1 mL has been collected, suction patient again before flushing catheter with normal saline. If secretions are extremely thick or tenacious, the catheter may flushed with a small amount (1 to 2 mL) of sterile normal saline. Allow patient to rest at least 1 minute between suctioning and replace oxygen delivery setup if necessary. Limit suctioning events to three times.	
___	___	___	12. When procedure is completed, turn off suction and disconnect catheter from suction tubing. Remove gloves inside out and dispose of gloves, catheter, and container with solution in proper receptacle.	
___	___	___	13. Suction the oral cavity and perform oral hygiene.	
___	___	___	14. Perform hand hygiene.	
___	___	___	15. Adjust patient's position. Auscultate chest to evaluate breath sounds.	
___	___	___	16. Label container with patient's name, time specimen was collected, any antibiotics administered within the last 24 hours, route of collection, and any other information required by institution policy.	
___	___	___	17. Record the time of suctioning, specimen sent, and the nature and amount of secretions. Also note the character of patient's respirations before and after suctioning. Also note on the laboratory request form any antibiotics administered in the last 24 hours.	

*Skill Checklists to Accompany Taylor's Clinical Nursing Skills:
A Nursing Process Approach*

Name _____   Date _____

Unit _____   Position _____

Instructor/Evaluator: _____   Position _____

Excellent	Satisfactory	Needs Practice	SKILL 14-21 **Using a Bag and Mask to Deliver Oxygen**	Comments
			Goal: To assist patient to maintain adequate oxygen saturation.	
___	___	___	1. Perform hand hygiene (if not crisis situation). Don disposable gloves. Put on goggles or safety glasses.	
___	___	___	2. Ensure that the mask is connected to the bag device, the oxygen tubing is connected to the oxygen source, and the oxygen is turned on. This may be done through visualization or by listening to the open end of the reservoir or tail; if air is heard flowing, the oxygen is attached and on.	
___	___	___	3. If possible, get behind patient's head of bed and remove the headboard of the bed. Slightly hyperextend patient's neck (unless contraindicated). If unable to hyperextend, use jaw thrust maneuver to open the airway.	
___	___	___	4. Place mask over patient's face with opening over oral cavity. If mask is teardrop shaped, the narrow portion should be placed over the patient's bridge of the nose.	
___	___	___	5. With dominant hand, place three fingers on patient's mandible, keeping head slightly hyperextended. Place thumb and one finger in C position around the mask, pressing hard enough to form a seal around patient's face.	
___	___	___	6. Using nondominant hand, gently and slowly (over 2 to 3 seconds) squeeze Ambu bag, watching chest for symmetric rise.	
___	___	___	7. Continue delivering breaths until patient's drive returns or until patient is intubated.	
___	___	___	8. Remove gloves and perform hand hygiene.	
___	___	___	9. Document the incident, including patient's respiratory effort before initiation of bag mask breaths, lung sounds, oxygen saturation, chest symmetry, and resolution of incident (i e, intubation or patient's respiratory drive returns).	

Skill Checklists to Accompany Taylor's Clinical Nursing Skills:
A Nursing Process Approach

Name _____   Date _____

Unit _____   Position _____

Instructor/Evaluator: _____   Position _____

Excellent	Satisfactory	Needs Practice	SKILL 15-1 **Starting an Intravenous Infusion**	Comments
			Goal: To provide a safe route for administration of intravenous therapy.	
___	___	___	1. Gather all equipment and bring to bedside. Check intravenous (IV) solution and medication additives with physician's order.	
___	___	___	2. Explain need for IV solution and procedure to patient.	
___	___	___	3. Perform hand hygiene. If using an anesthetic (numbing) cream, apply cream to a couple of potential insertion sites.	
___	___	___	4. Prepare IV solution and tubing.	
___	___	___	a. Maintain aseptic technique when opening sterile packages and IV solution.	
___	___	___	b. Clamp tubing, uncap spike, and insert into entry site on bag as manufacturer directs.	
___	___	___	c. Squeeze drip chamber and allow it to fill at least half way.	
___	___	___	d. Remove cap at end of tubing, release clamp and allow fluid to move through tubing. Allow fluid to flow until all air bubbles have disappeared. Close clamp and recap end of tubing, maintaining sterility of setup.	
___	___	___	e. If electronic device is used, follow manufacturer's instructions for inserting tubing and setting infusion rate.	
___	___	___	f. Apply label if medication was added to container. (Pharmacy may have added medication and applied label.) Label tubing with date and time tubing is hung.	
___	___	___	g. Place time-tape on container and hang IV on pole.	
___	___	___	5. Place patient in a low Fowler's position in bed. Place protective towel or pad under patient's arm.	
___	___	___	6. Select appropriate site and palpate accessible veins.	
___	___	___	7. If site is hairy and agency policy permits, clip a 2-inch area around intended entry site.	
___	___	___	8. Apply tourniquet 5 to 6 inches above venipuncture site to obstruct venous blood flow and distend vein. Direct	

Excellent	Satisfactory	Needs Practice		Comments
			SKILL 15-1 **Starting an Intravenous Infusion** *(Continued)*	

tourniquet ends away from entry site. Check to be sure radial pulse is still present.

___ ___ ___	9.	Ask patient to open and close his or her fist. Observe and palpate for a suitable vein. Try the following techniques if vein cannot be felt.	
___ ___ ___		a. Release tourniquet and have patient lower his or her arm below the level of the heart to fill the veins. Reapply tourniquet and gently tap over the intended vein to help distend it.	
___ ___ ___		b. Remove tourniquet and place warm moist compresses over intended vein for 10 to 15 minutes.	
___ ___ ___	10.	Don clean gloves.	
___ ___ ___	11.	If using intradermal lidocaine: Cleanse small area of possible insertion site with alcohol using a circular motion. Inject a small amount (0. 2 to 0. 3 mL) of lidocaine into the intradermal area. If using the numbing cream: Wipe cream off of insertion site. Cleanse the entry site with an antiseptic solution (alcohol swab) followed by antimicrobial solution (povidone iodine) according to agency policy. Use a circular motion to move from the center outward for several inches.	
___ ___ ___	12.	Use the nondominant hand, placed about 1 to 2 inches below entry site, to hold skin taut against vein. Avoid touching prepared site.	
___ ___ ___	13.	Enter skin gently with catheter held by the hub in the dominant hand, bevel side up, at a 10- to 30-degree angle. Catheter may be inserted from either directly over vein or from side of vein. While following the course of the vein, advance needle or catheter into vein. A sensation of "give" can be felt when needle enters vein.	
___ ___ ___	14.	When blood returns through lumen of needle or flashback chamber of catheter, advance either device $\frac{1}{8}$ to $\frac{1}{4}$ inch farther into vein. A catheter needs to be advanced until the hub is at the venipuncture site, but the exact technique depends on the type of device used.	
___ ___ ___	15.	Release tourniquet. Quickly remove protective cap from IV tubing and attach tubing to catheter or needle. Stabilize catheter or needle with nondominant hand.	
___ ___ ___	16.	Start solution flow promptly by releasing the clamp on the tubing. Examine the tissue around entry site for signs of infiltration.	

Excellent	Satisfactory	Needs Practice		Comments
			## SKILL 15-1 ## Starting an Intravenous Infusion *(Continued)*	
___	___	___	17. Secure the catheter with narrow nonallergenic tape ($\frac{1}{2}$ inch) placed sticky side up under hub and crossed over the top of the hub.	
___	___	___	18. Place sterile dressing over venipuncture site. Agency policy may direct nurse to use gauze dressing or transparent dressing. Apply tape to dressing if necessary. Loop tubing near entry site and anchor to dressing.	
___	___	___	19. Mark date, time, site, and type and size of catheter used for infusion on the tape. Anchor tubing.	
___	___	___	20. Remove all equipment and dispose of in proper manner. Remove gloves and perform hand hygiene.	
___	___	___	21. Anchor arm to an armboard for support, if necessary, or apply site protector or tube-shaped mesh netting over insertion site.	
___	___	___	22. Adjust rate of solution flow according to amount prescribed or follow manufacturer's directions for adjusting the flow rate on the infusion pump.	
___	___	___	23. Document the procedure and the patient's response. Chart time, site, device used, and solution.	
___	___	___	24. Return to check flow rate and observe for infiltration 30 minutes after starting infusion.	

Skill Checklists to Accompany Taylor's Clinical Nursing Skills:
A Nursing Process Approach

Name _____ Date _____

Unit _____ Position _____

Instructor/Evaluator: _____ Position _____

Excellent	Satisfactory	Needs Practice	SKILL 15-2 **Changing Intravenous Solution and Tubing**	Comments
			Goal: To safely maintain intravenous therapy using aseptic technique.	
____	____	____	1. Gather all equipment and bring to bedside. Check IV solution and medication additives with physician's order.	
____	____	____	2. Explain procedure and reason for changes to patient.	
____	____	____	3. Perform hand hygiene.	
			To Change Intravenous Solution	
____	____	____	4. Carefully remove protective cover from new solution container and expose bag entry site.	
____	____	____	5. Close clamp on tubing.	
____	____	____	6. Lift container off IV pole and invert it. Quickly remove spike from old IV container, being careful not to contaminate it.	
____	____	____	7. Steady new container and insert spike. Hang on IV pole.	
____	____	____	8. Reopen clamp on tubing, check drip chamber of administration set on tubing, and adjust flow.	
____	____	____	9. Label container according to agency policy. Record on Intake/Output record and document on chart according to agency policy. Discard used equipment in proper manner. Perform hand hygiene.	
			To Change Intravenous Tubing and Solution	
____	____	____	10. Follow Actions 1 through 4.	
____	____	____	11. Open administration set and close clamp on new tubing. Remove protective covering from infusion spike. Using sterile technique, insert into new container.	
____	____	____	12. Hang IV container on pole and squeeze drip chamber to fill at least halfway.	
____	____	____	13. Remove cap at end of tubing, release clamp, and allow fluid to move through tubing until all air bubbles have disappeared. Close clamp, attach adapter or connector (if necessary) to the end of the tubing, and recap end of tubing.	

Excellent	Satisfactory	Needs Practice		Comments
			SKILL 15-2 **Changing Intravenous Solution and Tubing** *(Continued)*	

To Change Tubing on a Short Extension Set

Excellent	Satisfactory	Needs Practice		Comments
___	___	___	14. Close the clamp on the existing IV tubing. Also close the clamp on the short extension tubing connected to the IV catheter in the patient's arm.	
___	___	___	15. Remove the current infusion tubing from the resealable cap on the short extension IV tubing. Using an alcohol wipe, swab the resealable cap and insert the new IV tubing into the cap. Proceed to 22.	

To Change Tubing Connected Directly
Into the Hub of the IV Access Catheter

Excellent	Satisfactory	Needs Practice		Comments
___	___	___	16. Follow Actions 10 through 13.	
___	___	___	17. Loosen tape at IV insertion site. Don clean gloves. Carefully remove dressing and tape.	
___	___	___	18. Place sterile gauze square under catheter hub.	
___	___	___	19. Place new IV tubing close to IV site and slightly loosen protective cap.	
___	___	___	20. Clamp old IV tubing. Steady the needle hub with nondominant hand until change is completed. Remove tubing with dominant hand using a twisting motion.	
___	___	___	21. Set old tubing aside. While maintaining sterility, carefully remove the covering or cap from the new administration set and insert sterile end of tubing into catheter hub. Twist to secure it; tape connection if necessary. Remove gauze square from under needle hub. Remove soiled gloves.	
___	___	___	22. Open the clamp on the IV tubing and check the flow.	
___	___	___	23. Reapply sterile dressing to site or tape catheter to patient according to agency protocol (see Skill 15-4).	
___	___	___	24. Regulate IV flow according to physician's order.	
___	___	___	25. Label IV tubing with date, time, and your initials. Label container and record procedure according to agency policy. Discard used equipment properly and perform hand hygiene.	
___	___	___	26. Record patient's response to IV infusion.	

Skill Checklists to Accompany Taylor's Clinical Nursing Skills:
A Nursing Process Approach

Name _____   Date _____

Unit _____   Position _____

Instructor/Evaluator: _____   Position _____

Excellent	Satisfactory	Needs Practice	SKILL 15-3 **Monitoring an Intravenous Site and Infusion**	
			Goal: To provide for safe delivery of prescribed intravenous fluids.	**Comments**
____	____	____	1. Monitor IV infusion several times a shift. More frequent checks may be necessary if medication is infused.	
____	____	____	a. Check physician's order for IV solution.	
____	____	____	b. Check drip chamber and time drops if IV is not regulated by an infusion control device.	
			c. Check tubing for anything that might interfere with flow. Be sure that clamp is in open position. Observe dressing for leakage of IV solution.	
____	____	____	d. Observe settings, alarm, and indicator lights on infusion control device, if one is being used.	
____	____	____	2. Inspect site for swelling, pain, coolness, or pallor at site of injection, which may indicate infiltration of IV. This necessitates removing IV line and restarting at another site.	
____	____	____	3. Inspect IV site for redness, swelling, heat and pain, which may indicate phlebitis is present; IV line will need to be discontinued and started at another site. Notify physician if you suspect phlebitis may have occurred.	
____	____	____	4. Check for local or systemic manifestations that indicate an infection is present at IV site. Discontinue the IV line and notify physician. Be careful not to disconnect IV tubing when putting on patient's hospital gown.	
____	____	____	5. Be alert for additional complications of IV therapy.	
____	____	____	a. Circulatory overload can result in signs of cardiac failure and pulmonary edema. Monitor input/output during IV therapy.	
____	____	____	b. Bleeding at the site is most likely to occur when IV therapy is discontinued.	
____	____	____	6. If possible, instruct patient to call for assistance if any discomfort is noted at IV site, solution container is nearly empty, flow has changed in any way, or pump alarm sounds.	
____	____	____	7. Document IV infusion, any complications of therapy, and patient's reaction to therapy.	

Skill Checklists to Accompany Taylor's Clinical Nursing Skills:
A Nursing Process Approach

Name _____ Date _____

Unit _____ Position _____

Instructor/Evaluator: _____ Position _____

Excellent	Satisfactory	Needs Practice	SKILL 15-4 **Changing an Intravenous Dressing**	Comments
			Goal: To control contamination of intravenous site and prevent introduction of microorganisms into bloodstream.	
			Peripheral	
___	___	___	1. Assess patient's need for dressing change.	
___	___	___	2. Gather equipment and bring to bedside.	
___	___	___	3. Explain procedure to patient.	
___	___	___	4. Perform hand hygiene. Don clean gloves.	
___	___	___	5. Place towel or disposable pad under arm with IV site. Carefully remove old dressing but leave tape that anchors IV needle or catheter in place. Discard in proper manner.	
___	___	___	6. Assess IV site for presence of inflammation or infiltration. If noted, discontinue and relocate IV line.	
___	___	___	7. Loosen tape and gently remove, being careful to steady catheter or needle hub with one hand. Use adhesive remover if necessary.	
___	___	___	8. Cleanse entry site with an alcohol swab using a circular motion moving from the center outward. Allow to dry. Follow with povidone-iodine swab using the same process.	
___	___	___	9. Reapply tape strip to needle or catheter at entry site.	
___	___	___	10. Apply sterile gauze or transparent polyurethane dressing over entry site. Remove gloves and dispose of properly. Perform hand hygiene.	
___	___	___	11. Secure IV tubing with additional tape if necessary. Label dressing with date, time of change, and initials. Check that IV flow is accurate and system is patent. Document findings.	
			Central Venous Access Device	
___	___	___	12. Follow Actions 1 to 5.	
___	___	___	13. Remove gloves and perform hand hygiene. Open dressing kit using sterile technique. If agency requires, nurse and patient should put on a mask.	
___	___	___	14. Put on sterile gloves.	

Changing an Intravenous Dressing *(Continued)*

Excellent	Satisfactory	Needs Practice		Comments
——	——	——	15. Cleanse the site according to agency policy such as using alcohol swabs, move in a circular fashion from the insertion site outward (1½ to 2-inch area). Allow to dry.	
——	——	——	16. Follow alcohol cleansing with povidone-iodine swabs using the same technique. Allow to dry.	
——	——	——	17 Reapply sterile dressing or securement device according to agency policy. Secure tubing or lumens to prevent tugging on insertion site.	
——	——	——	18. Note date, time of dressing change, size of catheter, and initial on tape or dressing.	
——	——	——	19. Discard equipment properly and perform hand hygiene.	
——	——	——	20. Record patient's response to dressing change and observation of site.	

Skill Checklists to Accompany Taylor's Clinical Nursing Skills:
A Nursing Process Approach

Name _____   Date _____

Unit _____   Position _____

Instructor/Evaluator: _____   Position _____

SKILL 15-5
Capping a Primary Line for Intermittent Use

Goal: To provide for intermittent venous access for delivery of prescribed medications.

Columns: Excellent | Satisfactory | Needs Practice | Comments

1. Gather equipment and verify physician's order. Fill lock end extension tubing with normal saline or heparin flush. Recap syringe for use in Action 10.
2. Explain procedure to patient.
3. Perform hand hygiene.
4. Assess IV site.
5. Clamp off primary line.

When Extension Tubing Is Present

6. Clamp the extension tubing if a clamp is present. Remove the primary IV tubing from the extension set and attach the lock or adapter device. Cleanse the cap of the lock of adapter device with an alcohol swab.
7. Unclamp the extension set and insert a saline or heparin flush syringe into the cap and flush the line according to agency policy. Reclamp the extension tubing and remove the syringe.
8. Use tape to secure the extension tubing. Proceed to 18.

When Connecting Directly to the Hub of the IV Access Catheter

9. Follow Actions 1 through 5.
10. Prime the lock of adapter device and extension set (if one is to be attached to the device) with normal saline. Clamp the extension set if one is being used.
11. Don clean gloves.
12. Place gauze 4" × 4" sponge underneath IV connection hub between IV catheter and tubing.
13. Stabilize hub of IV catheter with nondominant hand. Use dominant hand to quickly twist and disconnect IV tubing from the catheter. Discard it. Attach the primed lock or adapter device (or adapter device and extension set) to the IV catheter hub.
14. Cleanse cap with an alcohol wipe and unclamp the extension set (if used).

Capping a Primary Line for Intermittent Use
(Continued)

Excellent	Satisfactory	Needs Practice		Comments
___	___	___	15. Insert the syringe with blunt cannula or standard syringe and gently flush with saline or heparin flush as per agency policy. Remove syringe carefully and reclamp the extension tubing (if used).	
___	___	___	16. Remove gloves and dispose of them appropriately.	
___	___	___	17. Tape lock or adapter device (and extension tubing if used).	
___	___	___	18. Perform hand hygiene and ensure the patient is comfortable.	
___	___	___	19. Chart on IV administration record or medication Kardex per institutional policy.	

Skill Checklists to Accompany Taylor's Clinical Nursing Skills:
A Nursing Process Approach

Name _____ Date _____

Unit _____ Position _____

Instructor/Evaluator: _____ Position _____

Excellent	Satisfactory	Needs Practice	SKILL 15-6 **Administering a Blood Transfusion**	Comments
			Goal: To safely infuse blood or blood products into the venous circulation.	
___	___	___	1. Determine if patient knows reason for transfusion. Ask if patient has had a transfusion or transfusion reaction in the past.	
___	___	___	2. Explain procedure to patient. Make sure there is a signed consent for transfusion, if required by agency. Advise patient to report any chills, itching, rash, or unusual symptoms. If physician has ordered the patient to receive any premedication before receiving blood transfusion, administer the medication now.	
___	___	___	3. Perform hand hygiene and put on clean gloves.	
___	___	___	4. Hang container of 0.9% normal saline with blood administration set to initiate IV infusion and follow procedure for administration of blood.	
___	___	___	5. Start IV line with 18 or 19 gauge catheter, if not already present (see Skill 15-1). Keep IV line open by starting flow of normal saline.	
___	___	___	6. Obtain blood product from blood bank according to agency policy.	
___	___	___	7. Complete identification and checks as required by agency:	
___	___	___	a. Identification number	
___	___	___	b. Blood group and type	
___	___	___	c. Expiration date	
___	___	___	d. Patient's name	
___	___	___	e. Inspect blood for clots	
___	___	___	8. Take baseline set of vital signs before beginning transfusion.	
___	___	___	9. Start infusion of blood product.	
___	___	___	a. Prime in-line filter with blood.	
___	___	___	b. Start administration slowly (no more than 25 to 50 mL for the first 15 minutes). Stay with patient for first 5 to 15 minutes of transfusion.	

Excellent	Satisfactory	Needs Practice		Comments

SKILL 15-6

Administering a Blood Transfusion *(Continued)*

Excellent	Satisfactory	Needs Practice		Comments
—	—	—	c. Check vital signs at least every 15 minutes for the first half hour after start of transfusion. Follow the institution's recommendations for vital signs during the remainder of the transfusion.	
—	—	—	d. Observe patient for flushing, dyspnea, itching, hives, or rash.	
—	—	—	e. Never warm blood in a microwave. Use a blood-warming device, if indicated or ordered, especially with rapid transfusions through a central venous catheter.	
—	—	—	10. Maintain prescribed flow rate as ordered or as deemed appropriate by the patient's overall condition, keeping in mind the outer limits for safe administration. Assess frequently for transfusion reaction. Stop blood transfusion if you suspect a reaction. Quickly replace the blood tubing with new tubing and 0.9% sodium chloride. Notify physician and blood bank.	
—	—	—	11. When transfusion is complete, infuse 0.9% normal saline.	
—	—	—	12. Record administration of blood and patient's reaction as ordered by agency. Return blood transfusion bag to blood bank according to agency policy.	

Skill Checklists to Accompany Taylor's Clinical Nursing Skills:
A Nursing Process Approach

Name _____   Date _____

Unit _____   Position _____

Instructor/Evaluator: _____   Position _____

Excellent	Satisfactory	Needs Practice	SKILL 15-7 **Changing a PICC Line Dressing** **Goal:** To change dressing with patient remaining free of signs and symptoms of infection.	Comments
____	____	____	1. Gather equipment and verify physician's order (many times this will be a standing protocol).	
____	____	____	2. Explain procedure to the patient.	
____	____	____	3. Perform hand hygiene.	
____	____	____	4. If agency requires, apply a mask and have patient also put on a mask. Don clean gloves. Set up sterile field on area to be used. Have patient place arm in the middle of the sterile field. Open dressing kit using sterile technique and place on sterile towel.	
____	____	____	5. Assess PICC insertion through old dressing. Remove old dressing by lifting it distally and then working proximally. Remove gloves and dispose of properly. Put on sterile gloves.	
____	____	____	6. Starting at insertion site and continue in a circle, wiping off any old blood or drainage with a sterile alcohol wipe. Clean accordingly to agency policy such as using the alcohol swab sticks, one at a time, move in a circular fashion from the insertion site outward (2- to 3-inch area). Allow to dry.	
____	____	____	7. Follow alcohol cleansing with povidone-iodine swabs using the same technique. Allow to dry. If needed, you can then apply skin-protectant pad to this area, working from the insertion site out. Allow to dry.	
____	____	____	8. Reapply sterile dressing or securement device according to agency policy. Secure tubing or lumens to prevent tugging on insertion site.	
____	____	____	9. Clamp all lines of the PICC and remove injection caps. Cleanse the catheter ends with alcohol and then apply new injection caps. Tape the distal ends down securely.	
____	____	____	10. Note date, time of dressing change, size of catheter, and initials on tape or dressing.	
____	____	____	11. Discard equipment properly and perform hand hygiene.	
____	____	____	12. Record patient's response to dressing change and observation of site.	

Skill Checklists to Accompany Taylor's Clinical Nursing Skills:
A Nursing Process Approach

Name _____   Date _____

Unit _____   Position _____

Instructor/Evaluator: _____   Position _____

Excellent	Satisfactory	Needs Practice	SKILL 15-8 **Accessing an Implanted Port**	
			Goal: To access port with minimal to no discomfort to patient.	**Comments**
——	——	——	1. Gather equipment and verify physician's order (many times this will be a standing protocol).	
——	——	——	2. Explain the procedure to the patient.	
——	——	——	3. Perform hand hygiene.	
——	——	——	4. Raise the bed to a comfortable working height.	
——	——	——	5. Attach the blunt needles to the 10-mL syringes. Withdraw 10 mL of sodium chloride from the vial.	
——	——	——	6. Connect the intermittent injection cap to the extension tubing on the Huber needle. Attach the 10-mL syringe to the intermittent injection cap and flush the needle with tubing. Clamp the tubing. Remove the syringe from the injection cap.	
——	——	——	8. Open the kit using sterile technique. Don the mask and the first pair of sterile gloves. Set up your sterile field.	
——	——	——	7. If transparent dressing is in place, don clean gloves and gently pull it back, beginning with edges and proceeding around the edge of the dressing. Once dressing is removed, gently pull straight back on needle. Discard in appropriate receptacle amd remove gloves.	
——	——	——	8. Open the kit using sterile technique. Don the mask and the first pair of sterile gloves. Set up your sterile field.	
——	——	——	9. Cleanse according to agency policy. For example, using the alcohol swab sticks, wipe in a circular fashion from the insertion site outward (2- to 3-inch area). Use each swab once and discard. Allow to dry.	
——	——	——	10. Follow alcohol cleansing with povidone-iodine swabs using the same technique. Allow to dry.	
——	——	——	11. Locate the port septum by palpation. With your nondominant hand, hold the port stable, keeping the skin taut but without touching the port side.	
——	——	——	12. Visualize the center of the port. Push the Huber needle (noncoring 90 degree) to the skin into the portal septum until it hits the back of the port septum.	

Accessing an Implanted Port *(Continued)*

Excellent	Satisfactory	Needs Practice		Comments
___	___	___	13. Cleanse the injection cap with alcohol and insert the syringe with normal saline.	
___	___	___	14. Open the clamp and push down on the syringe plunger flushing the device with 3 to 5 mL of saline, while observing for fluid leak and/or infiltration. It should flush easily, without resistance.	
___	___	___	15. Pull back on the syringe plunger to aspirate for blood return. Aspirate only a few milliliters of blood; do not allow blood to enter syringe.	
___	___	___	16. Flush with the remainder of saline in syringe.	
___	___	___	17. Clamp the tubing, remove the syringe, and attach the heparin-filled syringe (if appropriate for the institution). Clamp the tubing while maintaining positive pressure on the syringe barrel at the end of the flush.	
___	___	___	18. Remove the syringe. If space exists between the skin and the needle, place a sterile folded 2″ × 2″ gauze pad in the space to support the needle. If using a "Gripper" needle, remove the gripper portion from the needle by squeezing the sides together and lifting off of the needle while holding the needle securely to the port with the other hand.	
___	___	___	19. Apply tape or Steri-Strips in a star-like pattern over the needle to secure it.	
___	___	___	20. Cover the entire needle and port with the transparent dressing, leaving the ports of the extension tubing uncovered for easy access.	
___	___	___	21. Remove gloves and discard. Perform hand hygiene.	
___	___	___	22. Label the dressing with the date, time, size needle used, and your initials, according to agency policy.	
___	___	___	23. Document the time, date, type and location of port, condition of skin at site, size needle used, the presence of a blood return, and any difficulties encountered.	

Skill Checklists to Accompany Taylor's Clinical Nursing Skills:
A Nursing Process Approach

Name _____   Date _____

Unit _____   Position _____

Instructor/Evaluator: _____   Position _____

Excellent	Satisfactory	Needs Practice	SKILL 15-9 **Deaccessing an Implanted Port**	
			Goal: To remove the needle with minimal or no discomfort to the patient	**Comments**
___	___	___	1. Gather equipment and verify physician's order (many times this will be a standing protocol).	
___	___	___	2. Explain the steps to the patient.	
___	___	___	3. Perform hand hygiene.	
___	___	___	4. Raise the bed to a comfortable working height.	
___	___	___	5. Don gloves.	
___	___	___	6. Begin to gently pull back transparent dressing, beginning with edges and proceeding around the edge of the dressing. Carefully remove all the tape that is securing the needle in place.	
___	___	___	7. Clean the injection cap and insert the saline filled syringe. Unclamp the catheter's extension tubing and begin to flush with a minimum of 10 mL normal saline.	
___	___	___	8. Remove the syringe and insert the heparin-filled syringe, flushing with 5 mL of heparin (100 μm/mL or agency's policy). Clamp the extension tubing while maintaining positive pressure on the barrel of the syringe. Remove the syringe.	
___	___	___	9. Secure the port on either side with the fingers of your nondominant hand. Grasp the needle/wings with the fingers of your dominant hand. Firmly and smoothly, pull the needle straight up at a 90-degree angle from the skin to remove it from the septum.	
___	___	___	10. Apply gentle pressure with the gauze to the insertion site. A Band-Aid may be applied over the port if any oozing occurs.	
___	___	___	11. Remove gloves and place bed in the lowest position. Make sure that the patient is comfortable before you leave the room.	
___	___	___	12. Perform hand hygiene.	
___	___	___	13. Document the date and time of deaccessing, the appearance of the site, ability to flush, and medication used to flush.	

Skill Checklists to Accompany Taylor's Clinical Nursing Skills:
A Nursing Process Approach

Name _____   Date _____

Unit _____   Position _____

Instructor/Evaluator: _____   Position _____

Excellent	Satisfactory	Needs Practice	SKILL 15-10 **Drawing Blood from a Central Venous Access Device**	Comments
			Goal: To obtain a blood specimen without injury to the patient, keeping central venous access device patent.	
____	____	____	1. Gather equipment and verify physician's order (many times this will be a standing protocol).	
____	____	____	2. Explain the steps to the patient.	
____	____	____	3. Perform hand hygiene.	
____	____	____	4. Raise the bed to a comfortable working height.	
____	____	____	5. Don gloves, mask, and protective eyewear.	
____	____	____	6. If IV fluids are infusing through the central venous access device (CVAD), stop the flow of fluids. Depending on facility policy, it could take up to 1 minute for standard IV fluids and up to 5 minutes for total parenteral nutrition, heparin, or any other solutions that may alter laboratory results.	
____	____	____	7. Position the patient for easy access to the CVAD, draping them if necessary to expose only the CVAD site.	
____	____	____	8. If more than one lumen is present, draw blood samples from the proximal lumen if possible.	
____	____	____	9. Cleanse the injection cap with alcohol and allow to air dry. *If blood is not being drawn with needless Vacutainer, continue to Action 17.*	
____	____	____	10. Place the Vacutainer adapter with the needleless cannula into the injection cap.	
____	____	____	11. Insert the discard tube into the Vacutainer and snap it into place. Fill the tube; 5 mL is the minimum for discard. Remove the discard tube from the sleeve and quickly insert and fill the desired collecting tubes.	
____	____	____	12. When the last tube of blood is obtained, remove the tube from the sleeve. Remove the Vacutainer cannula from the injection cap.	
____	____	____	13. Flush the lumen. If the lumen is not going to be used at present, flush with the appropriate saline and then heparin flush (if heparin is agency policy). If IV fluids are to be resumed, flush the lumen with 10 mL normal saline and resume IV fluids. Dispose of your equipment appropriately.	

Drawing Blood from a Central Venous Access Device
(Continued)

Excellent	Satisfactory	Needs Practice		Comments
——	——	——	14. Remove your gloves and place the bed in the lowest position. Make sure the patient is comfortable before you leave the room.	
——	——	——	15. Label the specimen tubes according to facility policy.	
——	——	——	16. Document the procedure according to agency policy and send the specimen to the laboratory.	
			If Blood Sample Is Drawn without the Use of a Vacutainer	
——	——	——	17. Clamp the lumen and insert a 10-mL syringe with a needleless cannula into the injection cap of the lumen. Unclamp the lumen and withdraw 5 mL of blood for discard. Clamp the lumen and remove the syringe and discard.	
——	——	——	18. Insert a 10- or 20-mL syringe with a needleless cannula into the injection cap, unclamp the lumen, and withdraw the blood needed for the studies. The total amount will depend on the amount needed for the ordered tests.	
——	——	——	19. Clamp the lumen and remove the syringe. Connect a blunt end needle to the syringe. Place blood in the appropriate tubes.	
——	——	——	20. Clear the port and then flush the lumen with the appropriate saline then heparin flush, according to facility policy.	
——	——	——	21. Dispose of your equipment appropriately. Remove your gloves. Place the bed in the lowest position.	
——	——	——	22. Label the specimen tubes according to facility policy.	
——	——	——	23. Document according to agency policy and send the specimen to the laboratory.	

Skill Checklists to Accompany Taylor's Clinical Nursing Skills:
A Nursing Process Approach

Name _____   Date _____

Unit _____   Position _____

Instructor/Evaluator: _____   Position _____

SKILL 16-1
Obtaining an Electrocardiogram

Goal: To obtain a cardiac tracing via machine without any complications.

Excellent	Satisfactory	Needs Practice		Comments
____	____	____	1. Place the electrocardiogram (ECG) machine close to the patient's bed and plug the power cord into the wall outlet.	
____	____	____	2. Perform hand hygiene. Check the patient's identification.	
____	____	____	3. As you set up the machine to record a 12-lead ECG, explain the procedure to the patient. Tell him that the test records the heart's electrical activity and it may be repeated at certain intervals. Emphasize that no electrical current will enter his body. Also, tell the patient that the test typically takes about 5 minutes.	
____	____	____	4. Have the patient lie supine in the center of the bed with his arms at his sides. Raise the head of the bed if necessary to promote his comfort. Expose the patient's arms and legs and drape appropriately. Encourage the patient to relax the arms and legs. If the bed is too narrow, place the patient's hands under his buttocks to prevent muscle tension. Also, use this technique if the patient is shivering or trembling. Make sure the feet are not touching the bed board.	
____	____	____	5. Select flat fleshy areas to place the electrodes. Avoid muscular and bony areas. If the patient has an amputated limb, choose a site on the stump.	
____	____	____	6. If an area is excessively hairy, clip it. Clean excess oil or other substances from the skin.	
____	____	____	7. Apply the electrode paste or gel or the disposable electrodes to the patient's wrists and to the medial aspects of his ankles. If using paste or gel, rub it into the skin. If using disposable electrodes, peel off the contact paper and apply the electrodes directly to the prepared site, as recommended by the manufacturer's instructions. Position disposable electrodes on the legs with the lead connection pointing superiorly.	
____	____	____	8. If using paste or gel, secure electrodes promptly after you apply the conductive medium. Never use alcohol or acetone pads in place of the electrode paste or gel.	

Excellent	Satisfactory	Needs Practice	SKILL 16-1 **Obtaining an Electrocardiogram** *(Continued)*	
				Comments
——	——	——	9. Connect the limb lead wires to the electrodes. The tip of each lead wire is lettered and color coded for easy identification. The white or RA lead wire goes to the right arm; the green or RL lead wire, to the right leg; the red or LL lead wire, to the left leg; the black or LA lead wire, to the left arm; and the brown or V_1 to V_6 lead wires, to the chest. Make sure the metal parts of the electrodes are clean and bright.	
——	——	——	10. Expose the patient's chest. Put a small amount of electrode gel or paste on a disposable electrode at each electrode position. Position chest electrodes as follows. • V_1: Fourth intercostal space at right sternal border • V_2: Fourth intercostal space at left sternal border • V_3: Halfway between V_2 and V_4 • V_4: Fifth intercostal space at midclavicular line • V^5: Fifth intercostal space at anterior axillary line (halfway between V_4 and V_6) • V_6: Fifth intercostal space at midaxillary line, level with V_4.	
——	——	——	11. Check to see that the paper speed selector is set to the standard 25 mm and that the machine is set to full voltage.	
——	——	——	12. If necessary, enter the appropriate patient identification data.	
——	——	——	13. Ask the patient to relax and breathe normally. Tell him to lie still and not to talk when you record his ECG.	
——	——	——	14. Press the AUTO button. Observe the tracing quality. The machine will record all 12 leads automatically, recording three consecutive leads simultaneously. Some machines have a display screen so you can preview waveforms before the machine records them on paper. Adjust waveform if necessary. If any part of the waveform extends beyond the paper when you record the ECG, adjust the normal standardization to half-standardization and repeat. Note this adjustment on the ECG strip because this will need to be considered in interpreting the results.	
——	——	——	15. When the machine finishes recording the 12-lead ECG, remove the electrodes and clean the patient's skin.	
——	——	——	16. After disconnecting the lead wires from the electrodes, dispose of or clean the electrodes, as indicated.	

Excellent	Satisfactory	Needs Practice		Comments
			SKILL 16-1 **Obtaining an Electrocardiogram** *(Continued)*	
___	___	___	17. Label the ECG recording with the patient's name, room number, and facility identification number, if not done by the machine. Also record the date and time as well as any appropriate clinical information on the ECG. Document the test's date and time as well as significant responses by the patient in the medical record.	

Skill Checklists to Accompany Taylor's Clinical Nursing Skills:
A Nursing Process Approach

Name _____   Date _____

Unit _____   Position _____

Instructor/Evaluator: _____   Position _____

Excellent	Satisfactory	Needs Practice	SKILL 16-2 **Applying a Cardiac Monitor**	
			Goal: To obtain a clear waveform that is free from artifact displayed on the cardiac monitor.	**Comments**
___	___	___	1. Gather all equipment and bring to bedside.	
___	___	___	a. Plug the cardiac monitor into an electrical outlet and turn it on to warm up the unit while preparing the equipment and the patient. For telemetry monitoring, insert a new battery into the transmitter. Be sure to match the poles on the battery with the polar markings on the transmitter case. Press the button at the top of the unit, test the battery's charge, and test the unit to ensure that the battery is operational.	
___	___	___	b. Insert the cable into the appropriate socket in the monitor.	
___	___	___	c. Connect the lead wires to the cable. In some systems, the lead wires are permanently secured to the cable. Each lead wire should indicate the location for attachment to the patient: right arm (RA), left arm (LA), right leg (RL), left leg (LL), and ground (C or V). These markings should appear on the lead wire—if it is permanently connected—or at the connection of the lead wires and cable to the patient. For telemetry, if the lead wires are not permanently affixed to the telemetry unit, attach them securely. If they must be attached individually, be sure to connect each one to the correct outlet.	
___	___	___	d. Then connect an electrode to each of the lead wires, carefully checking that each lead wire is in its correct outlet.	
___	___	___	2. Explain the procedure to the patient and provide privacy.	
___	___	___	3. Perform hand hygiene.	
___	___	___	4. Expose chest and determine electrode positions on the patient's chest, based on which system and lead being used. If necessary, clip the hair from an area about 10 cm in diameter around each electrode site. Clean the area with an alcohol pad and dry it completely to remove skin secretions that may interfere with electrode function.	

Excellent	Satisfactory	Needs Practice	SKILL 16-2 **Applying a Cardiac Monitor** *(Continued)*	**Comments**
____	____	____	5. Remove the backing from the pre-gelled electrode. Check the gel for moistness. If the gel is dry, discard it and replace it with a fresh electrode. Apply the electrode to the site and press firmly to ensure a tight seal. Repeat with the remaining electrodes to complete the three-lead or five-lead system.	
____	____	____	6. When all the electrodes are in place, check waveform for clarity, position, and size. To verify that the monitor is detecting each beat, compare the digital heart rate display with a palpated or auscultated count of the patient's heart rate. If necessary, use the gain control to adjust the size of the rhythm tracing and use the position control to adjust the waveform position on the monitor.	
____	____	____	7. Set the upper and lower limits of the heart rate alarm, based on unit policy. Turn the alarm on.	
____	____	____	8. For telemetry, place the transmitter in the pouch. Tie the pouch strings around the patient's neck and waist, making sure that the pouch fits snugly without causing the patient discomfort. If no pouch is available, place the transmitter in the patient's bathrobe pocket.	
____	____	____	9. To obtain a rhythm strip, press the RECORD key either at the bedside for monitoring or at the central station for telemetry. Label the strip with the patient's name and room number, date, time, and rhythm identification. Place the rhythm strip in the appropriate location in the patient's chart. Analyze strip as appropriate.	
____	____	____	10. Record the date and time that monitoring begins and the monitoring lead used in the medical record. Document a rhythm strip at least every 8 hours and with any changes in the patient's condition (or as stated by your facility's policy). Label the rhythm strip with the patient's name and room number, the date, and the time.	

Skill Checklists to Accompany Taylor's Clinical Nursing Skills:
A Nursing Process Approach

Name _____   Date _____

Unit _____   Position _____

Instructor/Evaluator: _____   Position _____

Excellent	Satisfactory	Needs Practice	SKILL 16-3 **Obtaining an Arterial Blood Sample**	
			Goal: To obtain a specimen with minimal discomfort and anxiety and without injury to the patient.	**Comments**
____	____	____	1. Assemble equipment. Label the syringe clearly with the patient's name and room number, the physician's name, the date and time of collection, and initials of the person performing the blood sample. If it is not already done, heparinize the syringe and needle. (See Skill 14-6.)	
____	____	____	2. Check the patient's identification. Explain the procedure to the patient. Confirm the patient's identity. Tell the patient you need to collect an arterial blood sample, and explain the procedure. Tell the patient that specimen will be obtained from the arterial line inserted.	
____	____	____	3. Perform hand hygiene and put on gloves.	
			Obtaining an Arterial Blood Sample From an Open System	
____	____	____	4. Assemble the equipment, taking care not to contaminate the dead-end cap, stopcock, and syringes. Turn off or temporarily silence the monitor alarms, depending on your facility's policy. (However, some facilities require that alarms be left on.)	
____	____	____	5. Locate the stopcock nearest the patient. Open a sterile 4 × 4 gauze pad. Remove the dead-end cap from the stopcock and place it on the gauze pad.	
____	____	____	6. Attach a syringe to obtain the discard sample into the syringe. Follow your facility's policy on how much discard blood to collect. In most cases, you will withdraw 5 to 10 mL through a 5- or 10-mL syringe.	
____	____	____	7. Turn the stopcock off to the flush solution. Slowly retract the syringe to withdraw the discarded sample. Then turn the stopcock halfway back to the open position to close the system in all directions. If you feel resistance, reposition the affected extremity and check the insertion site for obvious problems (such as catheter kinking). After correcting the problem, resume blood withdrawal.	
____	____	____	8. Remove the discard syringe and dispose of the blood in the syringe, observing standard precautions.	

Excellent	Satisfactory	Needs Practice	SKILL 16-3 **Obtaining an Arterial Blood Sample** *(Continued)*	Comments
——	——	——	9. Place the syringe for the laboratory sample in the stopcock, turn the stopcock off to the flush solution, and slowly withdraw the required amount of blood. For each additional sample required, repeat this procedure. If the physician has ordered coagulation tests, obtain blood for this sample from the final syringe.	
——	——	——	10. After you have obtained blood for the final sample, turn the stopcock off to the syringe and remove the syringe. Activate the fast-flush release (pigtail). Then turn off the stopcock to the patient and repeat the fast flush to clear the stopcock port.	
——	——	——	11. Turn the stopcock off to the stopcock port and replace the dead-end cap. Reactivate the monitor alarms. Attach needles to the filled syringes and transfer the blood samples to the appropriate containers, labeling them according to facility policy. Send all samples to the laboratory with appropriate documentation.	
——	——	——	12. Check the monitor for return of the arterial waveform and pressure reading.	
			Obtaining an Arterial Blood Sample From a Closed System	
——	——	——	13. Assemble the equipment, maintaining aseptic technique. Locate the closed-system reservoir and blood sampling site. Deactivate or temporarily silence monitor alarms. (However, some facilities require that alarms be left on.)	
——	——	——	14. Clean the sampling site with an alcohol swab.	
——	——	——	15. Holding the reservoir upright, grasp the flexures and slowly fill the reservoir with blood over a 3- to 5-second period. If you feel resistance, reposition the affected extremity and check the catheter site for obvious problems (such as kinking). Then resume blood withdrawal.	
——	——	——	16. Turn the one-way valve off to the reservoir by turning the handle perpendicular to the tubing. Using a syringe with attached cannula, insert the cannula into the sampling site. (Make sure the plunger is depressed to the bottom of the syringe barrel.) Slowly fill the syringe. Then grasp the cannula near the sampling site and remove the syringe and cannula as one unit. Repeat the procedure as needed to fill the required number of syringes. If the physician has ordered coagulation tests, obtain blood for those tests from the final syringe.	

SKILL 16-3

Obtaining an Arterial Blood Sample *(Continued)*

Excellent	Satisfactory	Needs Practice		Comments
___	___	___	17. After filling the syringes, turn the one-way valve to its original position, parallel to the tubing. Now smoothly and evenly push down on the plunger until the flexures lock in place in the fully closed position and all fluid has been reinfused. The fluid should be reinfused over a 3- to 5-second period. Then activate the fast-flush release.	
___	___	___	18. Clean the sampling site with an alcohol swab. Reactivate the monitor alarms. Using the blood transfer unit, transfer blood samples to the appropriate Vacutainer, labeling them according to facility policy. Send all samples to the laboratory with appropriate documentation.	
___	___	___	19. Follow actions 11 and 12 for an open system. Once the sample is obtained, check the syringe for air bubbles. If any appear, remove them by holding the syringe upright and slowly ejecting some of the blood onto a 2 × 2-inch gauze pad.	
___	___	___	20. Remove gloves and perform hand hygiene.	
___	___	___	21. Document time the sample was obtained, patient's temperature, arterial puncture site, amount of time pressure was applied to the site to control bleeding, and type and amount of oxygen therapy, if any, the patient was receiving.	

Name _____   Date _____

Unit _____   Position _____

Instructor/Evaluator: _____   Position _____

Comments

Excellent	Satisfactory	Needs Practice	SKILL 16-4 **Removing Arterial and Femoral Lines**	Comments
			Goal: To remove the line intact, without causing injury to the patient.	
___	___	___	1. Explain the procedure to the patient.	
___	___	___	2. Assemble all equipment. Perform hand hygiene. Observe standard precautions, including gloves and wearing personal protective equipment, for this procedure.	
___	___	___	3. Turn off the monitor alarms and then turn off the flow clamp to the flush solution. Carefully remove the dressing over the insertion site. Remove any sutures using the suture removal kit, making sure that all sutures have been removed.	
___	___	___	4. Withdraw the catheter using a gentle steady motion. Keep the catheter parallel to the artery during withdrawal.	
___	___	___	5. Immediately after withdrawing the catheter, apply pressure to the site with a sterile 4″ × 4″ gauze pad. Maintain pressure for at least 10 minutes (longer if bleeding or oozing persists). Apply additional pressure to a femoral site or if the patient has coagulopathy or is receiving anticoagulants.	
___	___	___	6. Cover the site with an appropriate dressing and secure the dressing with tape. If stipulated by facility policy, make a pressure dressing for a femoral site by folding four sterile 4 × 4 gauze pads in half, and apply the dressing. Cover the dressing with a tight adhesive bandage and then cover the femoral bandage with a sandbag. Maintain the patient on bedrest for 6 hours with the sandbag in place.	
___	___	___	7. Remove and properly dispose of gloves and personal protective equipment. Perform hand hygiene.	
___	___	___	8. Observe the site for bleeding. Assess circulation in the extremity distal to the site by evaluating color, pulses, and sensation. Repeat this assessment every 15 minutes for the first 4 hours, every 30 minutes for the next 2 hours, and then hourly for the next 6 hours.	
___	___	___	9. Document time the line was removed, how long pressure was applied, peripheral circulation, appearance of site, type of dressing applied, and the timed assessments.	

Skill Checklists to Accompany Taylor's Clinical Nursing Skills:
A Nursing Process Approach

Name _____ Date _____

Unit _____ Position _____

Instructor/Evaluator: _____ Position _____

SKILL 16-5
Performing Cardiopulmonary Resuscitation

Excellent **Satisfactory** **Needs Practice**

Goal: To maintain adequate function of the heart and lungs to sustain life.

Comments

___ ___ ___	1. Assess responsiveness; call for help and pull call bell if not responsive.	
___ ___ ___	2. Position the patient supine on his back and use the head tilt-chin lift maneuver to open the airway.	
___ ___ ___	3. Look, listen, and feel for air exchange.	
___ ___ ___	4. If no spontaneous breathing is noted, pinch the nose, while sealing patient's mouth with face shield or one-way valve mask (mouth and nose with Ambu bag), if available. If not available, seal mouth with your mouth.	
___ ___ ___	5. Instill two breaths, each lasting 2 seconds. Take a deep breath after providing each breath.	
___ ___ ___	6. If unable to ventilate or chest does not rise during ventilation, reposition head and reattempt to ventilate. Place in recovery position if breathing resumes. If still cannot ventilate, perform finger sweep and attempt five abdominal thrusts to remove obstruction. Repeat finger sweep and attempt to ventilate. Repeat this cycle as necessary	
___ ___ ___	7. Check carotid pulse and listen for spontaneous breathing.	
___ ___ ___	8. If no pulse, place backboard under patient (often the footboard of the patients bed). Position hands properly, with the heel of one hand approximately two fingerbreadths above the xyphoid process directly over the sternum, and then place the other hand directly on top of the first hand, keeping fingers above the chest.	
___ ___ ___	9. Perform 15 chest compressions at a rate of 100 per minute, counting "one and two and," up to 15, keeping elbows locked, arms straight, and shoulders directly over the hands.	
___ ___ ___	10. Give two rescue breaths after each set of 15 compressions. Do four complete cycles of 15 compressions and two ventilations.	
___ ___ ___	11. Reassess breathing and pulse after each set of four compression/breathing cycles.	

Excellent	Satisfactory	Needs Practice		Comments
			SKILL 16-5 **Performing Cardiopulmonary Resuscitation** *(Continued)*	
___	___	___	12. Continue cardiopulmonary resuscitation (CPR) until patient resumes spontaneous breathing and pulse, medical help arrives, or you are too exhausted to continue.	
___	___	___	13. Document the time you discovered the patient unresponsive and started CPR. Continued intervention such as by the code team will typically be documented on a code form, which identifies the actions and drugs provided during the code. Provide a summary of these events in the patient's medical record.	

Skill Checklists to Accompany Taylor's Clinical Nursing Skills:
A Nursing Process Approach

Name _____ Date _____

Unit _____ Position _____

Instructor/Evaluator: _____ Position _____

SKILL 16-6
Performing Emergency Defibrillation (Asynchronous)

Goal: To enable the patient to establish a spontaneous heart rate to sustain perfusion to vital organs with minimal patient complications.

Excellent	Satisfactory	Needs Practice		Comments
___	___	___	1. Assess the patient to determine whether he or she lacks a pulse. Call for help and perform cardiopulmonary resuscitation (CPR) until the defibrillator and other emergency equipment arrive.	
___	___	___	2. If the defibrillator has "quick-look" capability, place the paddles on the patient's chest. Otherwise, connect the monitoring leads of the defibrillator to the patient and assess his or her cardiac rhythm.	
___	___	___	3. Expose the patient's chest and apply conductive pads at the paddle placement positions. For anterolateral placement, place one paddle to the right of the upper sternum, just below the right clavicle, and the other over the fifth or sixth intercostal space at the left anterior axillary line. For anteroposterior placement, place the anterior paddle directly over the heart at the precordium, to the left of the lower sternal border. Place the flat posterior paddle under the patient's body beneath the heart and immediately below the scapulae (but not under the vertebral column).	
___	___	___	4. Turn on the defibrillator.	
___	___	___	a. If performing external defibrillation, set the energy level for 200 joules for an adult patient when using monophasic defibrillator. Use clinically appropriate energy levels for biphasic defibrillators.	
___	___	___	b. Charge the paddles by pressing the charge buttons, which are located either on the machine or on the paddles themselves (if pushing buttons on handles).	
___	___	___	c. Place the paddles over the conductive pads and press firmly against the patient's chest, using 25 pounds (11 kg) of pressure.	
___	___	___	5. Reassess the patient's cardiac rhythm.	
___	___	___	6. If the patient remains in ventricular fibrillation or pulseless ventricular tachycardia, instruct all personnel to stand clear of the patient and the bed, including yourself.	

Excellent	Satisfactory	Needs Practice		Comments
			SKILL 16-6 **Performing Emergency Defibrillation (Asynchronous)** *(Continued)*	

Excellent	Satisfactory	Needs Practice		Comments
___	___	___	7. Discharge the current by pressing both paddle charge buttons simultaneously.	
___	___	___	8. Leaving the paddles in position on the patient's chest, reassess the patient's cardiac rhythm and have someone else assess the pulse.	
___	___	___	9. If necessary, prepare to defibrillate a second time.	
___	___	___	a. Instruct someone to reset the energy level on the defibrillator to 200 to 300 joules or the biphasic energy equivalent.	
___	___	___	b. Announce that you are preparing to defibrillate and follow the procedure described above.	
___	___	___	10. Reassess the patient.	
___	___	___	11. If defibrillation is again necessary, instruct someone to reset the energy level to 360 joules or biphasic energy equivalent. Then follow the same procedure as before for a total of three shocks.	
___	___	___	12. If the patient still has no pulse after three initial defibrillations:	
___	___	___	a. resume CPR;	
___	___	___	b. give supplemental oxygen;	
___	___	___	c. begin administering appropriate medications such as epinephrine;	
___	___	___	d. also consider possible causes for failure of the patient's rhythm to convert, such as acidosis or hypoxia.	
___	___	___	13. If defibrillation restores a normal rhythm:	
___	___	___	a. Check the patient's central and peripheral pulses and obtain a blood pressure reading, heart rate, and respiratory rate.	
___	___	___	b. Assess the patient's level of consciousness, cardiac rhythm, breath sounds, skin color, and urine output.	
___	___	___	c. Obtain baseline arterial blood gas levels and a 12-lead electrocardiogram.	
___	___	___	d. Provide supplemental oxygen, ventilation, and medications, as needed.	
___	___	___	e. Check the patient's chest for electrical burns and treat them, as ordered, with corticosteroid or lanolin-based creams.	
___	___	___	f. Also prepare the defibrillator for immediate reuse.	

SKILL 16-6

Performing Emergency Defibrillation (Asynchronous)
(Continued)

Excellent	Satisfactory	Needs Practice		Comments
___	___	___	14. Document the procedure, including the patient's electrocardiographic rhythms both before and after defibrillation; the number of times defibrillation was performed; the voltage used during each attempt; whether a pulse returned; the dosage, route, and time of drug administration; whether CPR was used; how the airway was maintained; and the patient's outcome.	

Copyright © 2005 by Lippincott Williams & Wilkins. *Skill Checklists to Accompany Taylor's Clinical Nursing Skills: A Nursing Process Approach,* by Pamela Evans-Smith and Marilee LeBon.

Skill Checklists to Accompany Taylor's Clinical Nursing Skills:
A Nursing Process Approach

Name _____   Date _____

Unit _____   Position _____

Instructor/Evaluator: _____   Position _____

SKILL 16-7

Using an External (Transcutaneous) Pacemaker

Goal: To assist the patient to demonstrate an adequate heart rate that is capable of sustaining perfusion.

Excellent	Satisfactory	Needs Practice		Comments
____	____	____	1. If patient is responsive, explain the procedure to the patient and perform hand hygiene.	
____	____	____	2. If necessary, clip the hair over the areas of electrode placement. However, do not shave the area.	
____	____	____	3. Attach monitoring electrodes to the patient in the lead I, II, and III positions. Do this even if the patient is already on telemetry monitoring. If you select the lead II position, adjust the LL (left leg) electrode placement to accommodate the anterior pacing electrode and the patient's anatomy.	
____	____	____	4. Prepare the equipment.	
____	____	____	a. Put the patient cable into the electrocardiogram input connection on the front of the pacing generator. Set the selector switch to the MONITOR ON position.	
____	____	____	b. Note the electrocardiographic waveform on the monitor. Adjust the R-wave beeper volume to a suitable level and activate the alarm by pressing the ALARM ON button. Set the alarm for 10 to 20 beats lower and 20 to 30 beats higher than the intrinsic rate.	
____	____	____	c. Press the START/STOP button for a printout of the waveform.	
____	____	____	5. Apply the two pacing electrodes. Make sure the patient's skin is clean and dry to ensure good skin contact. Pull the protective strip from the posterior electrode (marked BACK) and apply the electrode on the left side of the back, just below the scapula and to the left of the spine.	
____	____	____	6. Apply the anterior pacing electrode (marked FRONT) which has two protective strips, one covering the gelled area and one covering the outer rim. Expose the gelled area and apply it to the skin in the anterior position, to the left side of the precordium in the usual V_2 to V_5 position. Move this electrode around to get the best waveform. Then expose the electrode's outer rim and firmly press it to the skin.	

Excellent	Satisfactory	Needs Practice	SKILL 16-7 **Using an External (Transcutaneous) Pacemaker** *(Continued)*	Comments
___	___	___	7. Prepare to pace the heart.	
___	___	___	a. After making sure the energy output in milliamperes (mA) is on 0, connect the electrode cable to the monitor output cable.	
___	___	___	b. Check the waveform, looking for a tall QRS complex in lead II.	
___	___	___	c. Next check the selector switch to PACER ON. Tell the patient that he or she may feel a thumping or twitching sensation. Reassure the patient that you will give him or her medication to tolerate the discomfort.	
___	___	___	d. Set the rate dial to 10 to 20 beats higher than the intrinsic rhythm. Look for pacer artifact or spikes, which will appear as you increase the rate. If the patient does not have an intrinsic rhythm, set the rate at 60.	
___	___	___	e. Slowly increase the amount of energy delivered to the heart by adjusting the OUTPUT mA dial. Do this until capture is achieved; you will see a pacer spike followed by a widened QRS complex that resembles a premature ventricular contraction.	
___	___	___	8. Increase output by 10%. Do not go higher because of the increased risk of discomfort to the patient.	
___	___	___	9. Document the reason for pacemaker use, time that pacing began, electrode locations, pacemaker settings, patient's response to the procedure and to temporary pacing, complications, and nursing actions taken. If possible, obtain a rhythm strip before, during, and after pacemaker placement; any time that pacemaker settings are changed; and whenever the patient receives treatment because of a complication due to the pacemaker.	
___	___	___	10. Assess the patient's vital signs, skin color, level of consciousness, and peripheral pulses.	
___	___	___	11. Perform a 12-lead electrocardiogram (ECG) and perform additional ECGs daily or with clinical changes.	
___	___	___	12. Continually monitor the ECG readings, noting capture, sensing, rate, intrinsic beats, and competition of paced and intrinsic rhythms. If the pacemaker is sensing correctly, the sense indicator on the pulse generator should flash with each beat.	

Skill Checklists to Accompany Taylor's Clinical Nursing Skills:
A Nursing Process Approach

Name _____ Date _____

Unit _____ Position _____

Instructor/Evaluator: _____ Position _____

Excellent	Satisfactory	Needs Practice	SKILL 17-1

SKILL 17-1
Caring for an External Ventriculostomy (Intraventricular Catheter Fluid-Filled System)

Goal: To assist the patient to maintain normal intracranial and cerebral perfusion pressures.

Comments

Excellent	Satisfactory	Needs Practice		
___	___	___	1. Explain procedure to patient. Review physician's order for specific information about parameters.	
___	___	___	2. Perform hand hygiene. Apply gloves if indicated.	
___	___	___	3. Assess patient for any changes in neurologic status.	
___	___	___	4. Assess height of ventriculostomy by ensuring that stopcock is at level of the foramen of Monro (outer canthus of the eye). Adjust height of system if needed. Move drip chamber to ordered height. Assess amount of cerebral spinal fluid in drip chamber if ventriculostomy is draining.	
___	___	___	5. Zero transducer. Turn stopcock off to the patient. Remove cap from transducer, being careful not to touch the end of the cap. Press and hold the calibration button on the monitor until the monitor beeps. Return cap to transducer. Turn stopcock off to drip chamber in order to obtain an ICP reading. After obtaining the reading, turn stopcock off to transducer.	
___	___	___	6. Move the ventriculostomy to prevent too much drainage, too little drainage, or inaccurate ICP readings.	
___	___	___	7. Care for the insertion site according to the institution's policy. Assess site for any signs of infection such as purulent drainage, redness, or warmth.	
___	___	___	8. Perform hand hygiene.	
___	___	___	9. Document the following information: amount and color of cerebrospinal fluid; ICP; CPP; pupil status; motor strength bilaterally; orientation to time, person, and place; level of consciousness; vital signs; pain; appearance of insertion site; and height of ventriculostomy.	

Skill Checklists to Accompany Taylor's Clinical Nursing Skills:
A Nursing Process Approach

Name _____ Date _____

Unit _____ Position _____

Instructor/Evaluator: _____ Position _____

SKILL 17-2
Caring for a Fiberoptic Intracranial Catheter

Excellent	Satisfactory	Needs Practice	**Goal:** To assist the patient to exhibit a normal intracranial and cerebral perfusion pressure.	Comments
____	____	____	1. Explain procedure to patient. Review physician's order.	
____	____	____	2. Perform hand hygiene.	
____	____	____	3. Assess patient for any changes in neurologic status.	
____	____	____	4. Assess insertion site for redness, drainage, or warmth.	
____	____	____	5. Assess ICP, MAP, and CPP at least hourly. Note ICP waveforms as shown on the monitor. Notify the physician if A or B waves are present.	
____	____	____	6. Perform hand hygiene.	
____	____	____	7. Document the following information: ICP; CPP; pupil status; motor strength bilaterally; orientation to time, person, and place; level of consciousness; vital signs; pain; and appearance of insertion site.	

Skill Checklists to Accompany Taylor's Clinical Nursing Skills:
A Nursing Process Approach

Name _____   Date _____

Unit _____   Position _____

Instructor/Evaluator: _____   Position _____

Excellent	Satisfactory	Needs Practice	SKILL 17-3 **Applying a Two-Piece Cervical Collar**	Comments
			Goal: To immobilize patient's cervical spine.	
___	___	___	1. Explain procedure to patient. Review physician's order.	
___	___	___	2. Perform hand hygiene and put on nonsterile gloves.	
___	___	___	3. Assess patient for any changes in neurologic status.	
___	___	___	4. Gently cleanse the face and neck with a mild soap and water. If patient has experienced trauma, inspect area for any broken glass or other material that could cut the patient or the nurse. Pat the area dry.	
___	___	___	5. While second person stabilizes cervical spine, measure the patient from the bottom of the chin to the top of the sternum to obtain height; measure around the neck to obtain circumference. Match the measurements to the manufacturer's recommended size chart.	
___	___	___	6. Slide flattened collar under the patient's head. The center of the collar should line up with the center of the patient's neck. Do not allow patient's head to move when passing the collar under the head.	
___	___	___	7. Place the front of the collar centered over the chin, while ensuring that the chin area fits snugly in the recess. Be sure that the front half of collar overlaps the back half. Secure Velcro straps on both sides.	
___	___	___	8. Check the skin under the cervical collar at least every 4 hours assessing for any signs of skin breakdown. Remove the top half of the collar daily and cleanse the skin under the collar. When collar is removed, have a second person immobilize the cervical spine.	
___	___	___	9. Remove gloves and perform hand hygiene.	
___	___	___	10. Document the condition of skin under the cervical collar, patient's level of consciousness, and patient's pain level.	

Skill Checklists to Accompany Taylor's Clinical Nursing Skills:
A Nursing Process Approach

Name _____   Date _____

Unit _____   Position _____

Instructor/Evaluator: _____   Position _____

Excellent	Satisfactory	Needs Practice	SKILL 17-4 **Logrolling a Patient**	Comments
			Goal: To keep the patient's spine in proper alignment, reducing risk for injury.	
___	___	___	1. Explain procedure to patient. Review physician's order.	
___	___	___	2. Perform hand hygiene.	
___	___	___	3. Position yourself on one side of the bed and have one or two assistants position on opposite side of bed. Place bed in flat position. Raise bed to height that is level with the nurses' hips. Place small pillow between the patient's knees.	
___	___	___	4. If patient is able to move arms, ask patient to cross his or her arms on chest. Roll or fanfold drawsheet to aid in obtaining a better grip (nurse and all assistants on opposite side of the bed). On the count of 3, all gently slide the patient to the side of the bed toward the nurse (the side opposite to which the patient will be turned). Ensure that sheet on side that patient is turning to is straightened and wrinkle free. Roll the drawsheet on side from which the patient is being turned.	
___	___	___	5. Grasp drawsheet at hip and shoulder level; have assistants on opposite side grasp drawsheet at areas above and below your area. On a predetermined signal, begin to turn the patient in one smooth motion trunk.	
___	___	___	6. Once turned, place a wedge or two pillows behind patient so that patient remains on the side and spine is in a straight line.	
___	___	___	7. Have assistant gently ease patient back onto pillows or wedge in one fluid-like movement.	
___	___	___	8. Stand at the foot of the bed and visualize the spinal column. The column should be straight, without any twisting or bending. Ensure that call bell and patient's telephone is within reach. Replace covers. Lower bed height.	
___	___	___	9. Perform hand hygiene.	
___	___	___	10. Document the condition of skin on patient's back, if any wounds or dressings are present and describe them, and patient's pain level.